Second Language Teaching

TOPICS IN LANGUAGE AND LINGUISTICS

Series Editors
Thomas A. Sebeok and Albert Valdman
Indiana University, Bloomington, Indiana

VOLUME 8

CONTEXTS OF COMPETENCE
Social and Cultural Considerations in Communicative Language Teaching
Margie Berns

THE DYNAMIC INTERLANGUAGE
Empirical Studies in Second Language Variation
Edited by Miriam R. Eisenstein

FRENCH AND CREOLE DISCOURSE, Second Edition
Edited by Albert Valdman

THE GRAMMAR OF DISCOURSE, Second Edition
Robert E. Longacre

ISSUES IN INTERNATIONAL BILINGUAL EDUCATION
The Role of the Vernacular
Edited by Beverly Hartford, Albert Valdman, and Charles R. Foster

LINGUISTICS AND LITERACY
Edited by William Frawley

LITERACY IN SCHOOL AND SOCIETY
Multidisciplinary Perspectives
Edited by Elisabetta Zuanelli sonino

THE RELATION OF THEORETICAL AND APPLIED LINGUSTICS
Edited by Olga Mišeska Tomić and Roger W. Shuy

Second Language Teaching

A View from the Right Side of the Brain

by

MARCEL DANESI
University of Toronto,
Canada

KLUWER ACADEMIC PUBLISHERS
DORDRECHT / BOSTON / LONDON

A C.I.P. Catalogue record for this book is available from the Library of Congress.

ISBN 1-4020-1488-0

Published by Kluwer Academic Publishers,
P.O. Box 17, 3300 AA Dordrecht, The Netherlands.

Sold and distributed in North, Central and South America
by Kluwer Academic Publishers,
101 Philip Drive, Norwell, MA 02061, U.S.A.

In all other countries, sold and distributed
by Kluwer Academic Publishers,
P.O. Box 322, 3300 AH Dordrecht, The Netherlands.

Printed on acid-free paper

Printed in the Netherlands

TABLE OF CONTENTS

PREFACE

At no other time in the history of education have teachers of languages been so knowledgeable about what to do in the classroom, or have had so many advanced tools at their disposal to help their students learn—from expertly-designed textbooks to technologically-sophisticated devices such as CD-ROMs. Yet, despite the many strides that teachers have made over the years, and notwithstanding the many sophisticated tools that they have at hand today, only a small fraction of students eventually achieve native-like proficiency at the end of a course of study. Why?

This question has bothered me throughout my professional life as a teacher of second languages. Disenchanted with existing methodologies, in the mid-1980s I ventured to seek insights from the domain of the neurosciences, thinking at the time that my theoretical adventure would probably turn out to be an unproductive one. To my surprise, it changed my view of learning drastically, allowing me to take charge of my classroom and to turn it into a veritable "field lab." Hence, the reason for this book. I have written it, simply, to communicate to my teacher colleagues the important pedagogical insights that I believe can be gained from an excursion into the neuroscientific domain.

Incidentally, my interest in the neurosciences brought me, in 1986, in contact with neuropsychologists and special education teachers working with brain-damaged children in Italy. From ensuing collaborative research on how to design teaching materials for such children, *Bimodality Theory* emerged—the view that the two primary modes of learning, the experiential and the analytical, must be activated in specific ways for such children (e.g. Danesi 1986 and D'Alfonso, Danesi, De Lellis, and Mastracci 1986). To my surprise, various Italian educators adopted Bimodality Theory shortly thereafter as a general framework for developing teaching curricula for handicapped children in school (D'Alonzo 1993). By the late 1980s, various second language teachers in Italy and North America started assessing the implications of Bimodality Theory critically for second language teaching in general (e.g. Lombardo 1988, Nuessel and Cicogna 1992, Pallotta 1993, Schenone 1994), and a number of doctoral students began investigating its principles empirically as potential constructs for second language acquisition (e.g. Arnò 1993, Curro 1995, Smor Forster 1995). Incidentally, when the term *bimodality* was proposed in 1986, I was not aware of the fact that it had already been in use among neuroscientists as a synonym for *Complementary Hemisphericity Theory* (e.g. Dunn 1985). I was also not cognizant of the fact that the term was employed by Laurence Ridge, a professor of mathematical education at the University of Toronto, five years earlier in 1981. Ridge's use of the term in that year was, to the best of my knowledge, the first time it was so utilized in the educational literature.

Bimodality Theory hardly stands alone as a "neuroscientifically-based proposal" for second language teaching. Interest among practitioners in brain research started, actually, in the late 1960s, right after linguist Eric Lenneberg published his widely-influential 1967 study, *The Biological Foundations of Language*, in which he put forward the hypothesis that there is a biologically-limited period for acquiring language that starts at birth and ends at adolescence. Neuroscientific research on the implications that Lenneberg's hypothesis had for the second language teaching profession at large was started almost immediately. Decades later, the time has come to ask ourselves if the fuss over the neurosciences has been worthwhile. Can knowledge about the brain truly inform not only the way we teach children with learning problems, but also the way we teach normal students in typical classroom situations? And what does it mean to say that a teaching approach is "brain-compatible?" These are the kinds of questions I will address in this book. However, from the outset I must make it clear that I will only *address* them, not attempt to *answer* them, simply because there is no empirical way to demonstrate that a specific teaching procedure is capable of activating a certain part of the brain—unless we put our students through a PET scan as we teach them something! And even if it could be shown that a certain part is activated, in response to a specific instructional stimulus, what would that truly mean, given that surprisingly little is known about the nature of the link between brain physiology and mental functions? Nevertheless, it is my cautious opinion that the foray into the neuroscientific domain on the part of practitioners in the last three decades or so has been a fruitful one. If nothing else, it has forced us to look more attentively and critically at the conditions we create in our classrooms and at the theoretical suppositions underlying new instructional practices or teaching syllabi proposed by educators. Good teaching is largely an art, and thus shaped mainly by hunches about what to do that come essentially from experience. But these hunches can certainly be confirmed or refined greatly by knowledge about how the brain acquires language.

I have used the manuscript of this book with prospective high school teachers of second languages over the last few years. Several of its parts are reworkings of previously-published research, supported by various grants from the Social Sciences and Humanities research Council of Canada, to whom I am very grateful. These have been integrated into the present book without hopefully compromising its coherence. Lacking from the present treatment are the actual data and the analyses of the studies that support Bimodality Theory. Readers can examine these first-hand themselves by consulting the relevant references in the bibliography provided at the back.

This volume has not been designed as a "research monograph," but rather as a "neuroscientific essay" on the principles that in my opinion should form the basis of "informed" second language teaching. I have written it with a particular *view* in mind—a *view* "from the right side of the brain," so to speak. Therefore, although it has all the typical features of other methodology books, such as historical accounts of language teaching trends, synopses of the main learning theories, overviews of suitable techniques, etc., it provides a different framework for *viewing* them.

I must warn readers from the outset about what not to expect from this book. First, they will not find in it an in-depth treatment of *neuroscience* or *neurolinguis-*

tics proper. Relevant introductory manuals in these fields are listed in the bibliography at the back, which contains not only cited works, but also those dealing generally with neuroscience and second language learning and teaching. Second, readers should not expect to find a prescription in it of how to teach a language methodically. Brain research is useful only in providing *insights,* not overarching *solutions*. I will, however, discuss in some detail the implications that Bimodality Theory would seem to hold in store for language teaching practices. Whether readers agree or disagree with any or all of my comments, is beside the point of this book. My only hope is that they will be stimulated by it to know more about brain-compatible second language teaching. That and that alone will have made its writing worthwhile, for I believe that such knowledge can form the basis for developing pedagogy that will lead to enhanced learning outcomes for students today.

I would like to thank my students at the Ontario Institute for Studies in Education, the University of Toronto, the University of Perugia, and the University of Lugano. Their critical responses to Bimodality Theory, along with the many enthusiastic classroom discussions that I have had with them over the years, have encouraged me to write this manual for a broader audience. A special thanks goes out to those teachers and researchers who have become interested in Bimodality Theory, and who have become both its most enthusiastic supporters and its most effective critics. The many suggestions they have made to me over the years have been incorporated into this book. I owe a special debt of gratitude to the late Thomas A. Sebeok and to Professor Albert Valdman of Indiana University for the unwavering support they have always given to my ideas, and for inviting me to synthesize them in book form. Most of the content of this book has, in any case, been inspired by their truly pivotal work in linguistics, education, and semiotics. As a graduate student at the University of Toronto in the late 1960s I came under the spell of their writings. These have left an indelible mark on my own research and writing.

Last but not least, I must thank my family, Alexander, Sarah, Lucia, Danila, Christopher, and Danilo for having been tolerant and patient with me as I worked on this book. I know I have been grumpy and absent-minded in the process. I dedicate this book to them.

Marcel Danesi
University of Toronto, 2003

CHAPTER 1
THE SECOND LANGUAGE TEACHING DILEMMA

They spell it Vinci and pronounce it Vinchy; foreigners always spell better than they pronounce.

Mark Twain (1835-1910)

Introduction

The 1880s constitute a significant period in the history of language education. That was the decade in which a group of teachers initiated a grassroots movement, known as the *Reform Movement*, that changed the course of language teaching in a radical way. The objective of those educational "reformers" was to tackle head-on the conceivable reasons why students of languages at school seemed invariably to experience so many difficulties and, by the end of a course of study, to achieve such low levels of proficiency. Why is it, they asked, that language learning in a classroom environment is such a challenging and generally unproductive experience, especially when compared to how easily and *naturally* the native language is acquired during infancy and childhood? The reformers believed that this predicament was not connected, in any way whatsoever, to any diminished ability to learn languages after childhood, but rather to the archaic language teaching method being used in the schools at the time—the so-called *Grammar-Translation Method*.

Is there anything, they asked, that could be done *in the classroom* to make language learning less of a struggle, and more comparable to how the native language is acquired? The reformers turned to the then-fledgling sciences of linguistics and psychology. Their aim was to extract pedagogical principles from the scientific research on both *language* by linguists and on the *learner* by psychologists and then convert these into a *scientifically-designed* method that they hoped would tap into the students' innate language-learning resources in a productive way. The reformers presented and argued their case persuasively to their fellow teachers. Their argument was so compelling that it has left a legacy to this day. In fact, thanks to the Reform Movement it is virtually impossible to think of second language teaching as anything but a scientifically-designed form of instruction grounded in some theory of learning.

Over a century and a quarter later, however, the reformist paradigm has hardly lived up to the expectations it raised at the outset. Students everywhere continue to complain about the effort it takes to learn a new language and about the insufficient levels of proficiency they attain, *no matter how hard they try or how competent the teacher is.* This raises a fundamental question: Was the reformist paradigm a misguided one? Many now believe that it was. I do not. Theoretically-informed language teaching *can* make a difference, even if within certain limits. The main objective of this book is, in effect, to revisit the dilemma faced by the reformers and the *theory-into-practice* paradigm they established to resolve it. Like the reformers, I will also tackle the dilemma by turning to a scientific domain for insights—the neuroscientific one. However, before doing so, it is necessary to establish a historical frame-of-reference that will allow me to discuss the dilemma and the paradigm in a meaningful way. That is the goal of this opening chapter.

Throughout this chapter and book I will use certain terms and abbreviations in specific ways. These are now standard in professional discussions of second language teaching. They are listed in the glossary at the back for convenience. The term *native language* (NL) refers to the language (or languages) acquired during infancy and childhood in a *natural* context. The term *first language* is also used in the literature as a synonym for native language. The term *second language* (SL) refers to any language learned after the NL. In this book SL will be used exclusively to designate any language learned formally in school after childhood. In this latter sense, the terms *foreign language* and *target language* are also used interchangeably in the professional literature. The term *native language acquisition* (NLA), rather than *native language learning*, is the one preferred today by most linguists and developmental psychologists. Analogously, the term *second language acquisition* (SLA), rather than *second language learning*, is the preferred one, and will thus be used in this book as well.

The term *methodology* refers to the practice of devising pedagogical practices, techniques, learning materials, etc. based on both the relevant research on learning and the insights of practitioners. The word *syllabus* refers to the organization of a course, or program of study, in terms of a specific view of learning: e.g. a *structural syllabus* would specify *which* structures of pronunciation, grammar, etc. are to be taught and in *what* sequence they are to be taught. The term *method* designates a pre-set, fixed way of designing a syllabus, carrying out procedures in a classroom, and preparing learning materials; *approach*, on the other hand, refers to a more flexible way of doing the same kinds of things. The word *technique* denotes a specific procedure for carrying out some pedagogical task or instructional objective. Finally, *input* refers to the linguistic information to which a learner is exposed and from which he/she is supposed to learn something specific; while *intake* refers to the actual information the learner takes away from the input and is able to store into long-term memory.

The SLT Dilemma

Ever since the Reform Movement, the teaching of SLs has been informed by theories and findings coming out of psychology and linguistics. This interplay between research and practice has produced teachers who are among the most skilled and knowledgeable in the entire field of education. As we enter the first decade of the twenty-first century it is, in fact, difficult to think of the SL classroom in high school, college, or university as anything but a highly advanced learning environment. So, why is there, despite the apparent sophistication, still so much debate going on in scholarly journals, and among practitioners at conferences and meetings, about what to do to make SLA effective and student discourse more native-like? The recent literature has even rekindled an old debate. Should we continue to focus on developing in the learner a functional knowledge of the target language? Or, should we return to the deployment of age-old techniques designed to help learners develop a conscious control of grammatical structure?

This debate has been re-ignited, no doubt, because teachers continue to be frustrated by the inability of their students to speak in ways that reflect how native speakers of the target language do and because it persistently takes them so much time and effort to produce even the simplest of sentences, let alone entire discourses. The nagging and enduring *second language teaching* (SLT) *Dilemma* can be articulated as follows:

> Why is it that, despite considerable research on second language acquisition in classroom environments in the last 125 years, and despite the many pedagogical advancements that such research has made possible, students rarely achieve high levels of proficiency, no matter how long they have been studying a language and no matter how they have been taught the language?

Some teachers now reject the reformist theory-into-practice paradigm completely, since no scientifically-designed pedagogical method has ever proven itself to be universally effective. As Selinker (1972) descried a little while back, barely 5% of all language students exposed to classroom pedagogy eventually achieve native-like proficiency in the SL, no matter what kind of instruction they may have received. The vast majority of students, Selinker lamented, were going to have to be satisfied with learning approximations of the SL. Many of those who reject the reformist paradigm generally tend to seek other ways to deliver SL training—e.g. through immersion training or through a "languages across the curriculum" approach (whereby the SL is used by students as a tool to learn other school subjects). Both solutions, incidentally, have ancient roots. In many parts of the ancient world, selected young learners were sent regularly to do their language learning *in loco*, i.e. in the actual societies where they would be later stationed. From their "immersion experience," it was believed they could learn to speak the foreign language effortlessly and naturally. And, it was the Romans who introduced the "languages across the curriculum" approach, teaching Greek to their children within their own school system, thus establishing one of the earliest models of early childhood bilingual education. In the first years of life, a Roman child would be entrusted to a Greek-speaking slave or nurse so that he/she could be exposed naturally to the language. When the child reached school age he/she would then be taught the curriculum in the two languages—at first by a Greek *grammaticós* (grammar teacher) and a Latin *ludi magister* (task/game master), and a little later by a Greek *rhetor* (teacher of rhetoric) and a Latin *orator* (teacher of oratory) (Titone 1968: 6).

Yet, despite the many successes that have been documented for contemporary immersion and languages-across-the-curriculum approaches, the search for appropriate classroom pedagogy goes on relentlessly nonetheless. The SLT Dilemma is a challenge from which teachers simply refuse to shy away. The reformist dream of turning the classroom into an effective learning environment is alive and well in many professional quarters, as teachers today continue to seek some practical theoretical framework that will allow them to understand: (1) *what* to do in certain situations, (2) *when* to do it, (3) *how* to do it, and (4) *what* to expect realistically from the students. The view adopted in this book is that the insights and techniques to make SLA effective *in classroom environments* already exist. I agree with many of my colleagues that what is needed is a "practical theory" that can help us synthesize, coordinate, and apply what we now know in ways that reflect both teacher and student expectations. However, before suggesting what such a theory would entail, it is necessary, as mentioned above, to step back and take a contemporary birds-eye view at how the Dilemma has been tackled in the past and at what the general research on language acquisition tells us.

The "Method Response"

For most of the twentieth century the standard "game plan" for tackling the SLT Dilemma was a relatively straightforward one. It consisted, essentially, in converting the scientific research on language and learning into a teaching *method*. The implicit assumption was that the level of SL proficiency achieved by *most of the students* was proportional to the degree of accuracy with which the method reflected the relevant research implications, *regardless of who was doing the teaching*. As mentioned, this game plan originated in the 1880s, when language educators made the first serious attempts to model instructional practices after specific theories of learning. The central objective of the Reform Movement was to unify pedagogical practices by developing an appropriate *curriculum* or *syllabus* (as it eventually came to be known) as the consolidating framework for these practices.

Grammar-Translation Pedagogy

Motivated by the premise that effective classroom instruction should be carried out according to psychologically-valid principles of learning, the Reform Movement emerged in reaction to the prevailing eighteenth and nineteenth century practice known as *Grammar-Translation* (GT) pedagogy. The main characteristic of the *Grammar-Translation Method* (GTM), as it came subsequently to be known, was the explicit teaching of grammatical rules that learners were expected to memorize and then apply as best they could to translation tasks. The GTM traced its roots to the medieval and early Renaissance periods, when only Latin and Greek were deemed worthy of formal study in European schools. The study of vernacular languages was tied to a practical need, and was assumed, as in the ancient world, to be best accomplished through immersion learning, which McArthur (1983: 94) characterizes as the "marketplace" approach to SLA—the place where words have impact and get results.

Latin and Greek were taught in a straightforward *deductive* way: teachers first presented a rule of grammar, after which they assigned oral and written translation tasks to students so that their ability to apply the rule could be assessed. As the social and educational functions of Latin came to be assumed more and more by vernacular languages in the sixteenth century (from Latin *vernaculus* "domestic, native"), the formal study of those languages started to take on increasing society-wide importance. It was decided that the same basic GT approach used to teach Latin and Greek could be adopted to teach the vernacular languages. From the outset, controversy surrounded this decision. Educators such as Guarino Guarini (1374-1460), St. Ignatius of Loyola (1491-1556), and Wolfgang Ratke (1571-1635) argued that GT pedagogy ignored *how* languages were learned by children and by those who acquired them effortlessly in the marketplace. In the seventeenth century, Jan Komensky, the Protestant bishop of Moravia, better known by his Latin name Comenius (1592-1670), made a truly persuasive case against the GT view of language instruction. He claimed that students learned best when they had to decipher and produce *dialogues* scripted to reflect real life. From the study of such dialogues, he suggested, they could easily induce the appropriate grammatical rules on their own.

In the school systems of the seventeenth and eighteenth centuries, however, GT pedagogy prevailed. It simply had too much tradition behind it and, moreover, it was a very easy method to implement in classrooms, given its straightforward deductive approach, which put the onus of learning directly on the students' shoulders. The main features of GT pedagogy were as follows.

- The instructor taught grammatical rules explicitly in the learner's NL. The rules were derived from classical models of grammar, rather than from any scientific analysis of the structure of the vernacular language.
- The teacher compared the new items of SL grammar and vocabulary to corresponding NL items.
- The students were required to memorize the grammatical rules as well as the vocabulary used to illustrate them.
- The students were then assigned oral and written translation tasks, ranging from single words to the entire translation of texts written in either the SL or the NL.
- The texts came with bilingual glossaries and annotations, which the students were expected to consult as they carried out their translation tasks.
- Mechanical exercises were also used, so that the students could reinforce grammatical knowledge (e.g. inflecting nouns, conjugating verbs, etc.).

Essentially, the typical nineteenth-century student of languages had to first learn a system of abstract rules of grammar and then apply them to specific translation tasks. The latter were considered to be the means through which the learner tested, reinforced, and expanded his/her developing knowledge of the target language. But the GTM rarely produced satisfactory results. The problem was, simply, that most students did not possess the grammatical background knowledge that they were expected to bring to the learning tasks at hand. And even those who were adept at memorizing rules and applying them to translation problems successfully manifested difficulties in the other domains of the SL—especially in oral fluency.

The Direct Method

Like Comenius before them, reformers such as Gouin (1880) and Viëtor (1886) saw the emphasis on grammar training as misguided. Moreover, they argued that deductive pedagogy was clearly not the best way to help students of *all backgrounds and abilities* learn a new language. The reformers thus turned their attention to the scientific domain for insights. Their decision to do so was influenced by five crucial events:

- Linguistics was emerging at the time as a scientific discipline. This gave rise to a new scientific perception of SL grammar.
- Psychology had been established a few decades earlier as a scientific enterprise. The reformers claimed that teachers should use the findings of psychologists on language learning to guide them in selecting what was to be taught and when to teach it in a more opportune manner.
- The Modern Language Association of America was founded in 1883 and the Modern Language Association of Great Britain in 1889, both of which focused attention on the importance of the teaching method itself in enhancing learning outcomes for *all types* of learners.
- The International Phonetic Association was established in 1886, raising awareness about the importance of accurate pronunciation in language learning.
- National languages came to play increasingly important roles on the stage of world relations after the Industrial Revolution. This led to a practical need on the part of the average person to learn foreign languages in school. The reformers wanted to turn this need into an achievable goal for all, not just for those with a talent for languages.

This new *Zeitgeist* led to the construction of the first ever "scientific" teaching method, called the *Direct Method* (DM), in the 1880s. The DM immediately attained official recognition in France and Germany, despite misgivings about its overall objectives on the part of several of the reformers. It was subsequently adopted *en masse* in England and the United States. Its main features were as follows:

- All instruction and classroom activities were carried out in the target language from the very outset. For this reason, it was considered preferable for the teacher to be a native speaker of the language, so that he/she could provide native input constantly.
- Utilization of the NL was discouraged. The new vocabulary was imparted *directly* through actions, gestures, pictures, objects, etc. (hence the term *Direct Method*).
- Every lesson began with listening and imitation activities revolving around a dialogue. To ensure that these were learning-effective and appropriate, uniformly-constructed textbooks were introduced as the basis of instruction (Richards and Rodgers 1986: 7-8). These contained

the dialogues and follow-up exercises arranged in order of increasing complexity.

- Pattern practice exercises followed, from which the learner was expected to induce the relevant rules of grammar inherent in them.
- Reading and writing instruction and practice followed this initial oral learning stage. From this the chronological teaching of the four skills was introduced into SLT: *listening-speaking-reading-writing*.

The DM—known vicariously as the *Phonetic Method* or the *Reform Method*—was, in actual fact, the more widely-used of the so-called *Natural Methods*, which included the commercially-profitable ones of Saveur and Berlitz, designed more for individualized study than for classroom learning (Titone 1968: 100-101, Richards and Rodgers 1986: 9-10). Although most of its practices had historical parallels—pattern practice drills, for instance, were traceable to the substitution tables of sixteenth- and seventeenth-century grammars, and pedagogically-designed situational dialogues to the writings of Comenius—never before were they organized so systematically and coherently. The way in which the DM interrelated the language, the teacher, the learner, the situation, and the actions that took place within the classroom changed SLT in a radical way. Indeed, many of the DM's suggestions and techniques continue to be used to this day (whether or not it is known) in a variety of guises and disguises.

The techniques that characterized the DM were designed to simulate the inductive processes involved purportedly in NLA. The SLA = NLA view on which the DM was constructed became, *ipso facto*, the first ever "second language learning theory." Predictably, it generated controversy almost from the outset. Henry Sweet (1899), for instance, argued that adults, unlike children, brought previous language experiences to their learning tasks. Sweet also warned against the assumption that *all students* learned in the same way—through induction. A little later, the British educator Harold Palmer (1917, 1921, 1922) expressed similar reservations about the *all-or-nothing* perspective adopted by adherents of the DM. The students' diverse backgrounds and motivations for studying a language, Palmer argued, warranted the need for instructional flexibility. Rather than develop a single, standard view of language learning, it was better to have a "set of principles," Palmer (1917: 8) suggested, that reflected the anecdotal experiences of teachers and students, not only the findings of psychologists and linguists, especially since the SLA process was characterized by *stages*, which were reached at different times by different types of learners. Palmer thus recommended that new items of SL grammar and vocabulary be introduced and taught gradually and in accordance with what the students could actually absorb—not in a pre-fixed, uniform way.

The critiques of Sweet and Palmer were, in hindsight, high theoretical peaks of a groundswell of anti-reformist sentiment that started taking root at the turn of the twentieth century. The DM had shown its main weakness through actual usage—it was simply too dogmatic and inflexible in its overall view of SLA, ignoring the "facts of variability" in student learning abilities, not to mention in teacher abilities and preferences. By the early 1920s, disenchantment with the DM had reached a critical mass. It was abandoned *en masse* shortly thereafter.

The Reading and Oral Methods

With the demise of the DM a new debate was ignited between those who continued to subscribe to its basic *inductivist* approach and those who wanted to return to the *deductivist* approach of the GTM. From this debate, two new methods—the *Reading* and the *Oral Methods*—emerged. The former grew out of the widely-held view in the 1920s that the only realistically-attainable goal in a non-immersion learning environment was reading comprehension, not native-like oral fluency. Like the GTM, the Reading Method stressed the role of grammar instruction and translation tasks. But unlike the GTM, it emphasized accurate pronunciation (which it regarded as an indispensable aid to comprehension) and the need to formulate explanations of grammar in terms of a more scientific analysis of the target language. It also introduced into the general practice of SLT the highly useful notions of controlled vocabulary learning and of graded readers. The main features of the Reading Method can be summarized as follows:

- Grammar was taught in the NL, and geared towards the decipherment of a given reading.
- The vocabulary to be learned was taken from the readings.
- Translation exercises were used extensively, along with pattern practice exercises. These were, however, tied to the contents of the readings.
- The reading texts were sequenced according to increasing syntactic and stylistic complexity.
- Proper pronunciation of words and sentences was emphasized throughout a course of study.

Versions of the Reading Method continue to have many adherents to this day because, as a deductivist method, it makes few demands on teachers, and therefore continues to have considerable appeal in situations where the primary goal of SL study is the reading of literary texts, as in university language and literature programs. What Richards and Rodgers (1986: 5) pointed out in the mid-1980s about deductivist approaches continues to ring true today. They are widely popular, even though they have no advocates, because they constitute a form of instruction "for which there is no theory."

The *Oral Method* (also called the *Situational Method*) was developed by British linguists in the 1930s. It was seen at the time as an attempt to revive the DM in an updated fashion. Among the techniques it proposed—many of which continue to be used today by many textbook authors and syllabus designers—the following gave the Oral Method its essential character:

- It stressed a sequential approach to vocabulary, starting with the teaching of the concrete lexical items used in everyday situations, and progressing gradually to the teaching of abstract items used primarily for rhetorical or specialized purposes.
- It organized its grammatical syllabus in a similar way by sequencing the structures of the SL to be taught in order from simple to complex.

- It introduced the new material to be learned orally (hence the name *Oral Method*).
- It claimed that reading and writing skills were to be taught after it could be determined that students had attained a sufficient level of lexical and grammatical competence.
- It insisted on the exclusive use of the SL in the classroom.
- It introduced the idea of the "situational practice" of new notions and structures, thus foreshadowing the so-called contextualized language teaching techniques of the 1980s and 1990s.

The Oral Method's practice of introducing vocabulary early on to reflect everyday real-life situations made it highly popular with teachers and learners alike (Halliday, McIntosh and Strevens 1964: 38). Its grammatical syllabus, which graded structures from simple to complex, came a little later to be known as the *structural syllabus*. This syllabus has remained virtually intact to this day, especially as a guide to the preparation of textbooks.

The Audiolingual Method

Neither the Reading nor the Oral Method ever really attracted the same level of followers that the DM did, perhaps because neither was the product of a "grassroots movement," as was the DM. And, neither one ever generated the same kind of enthusiastic expectations that the DM did. However, by the early 1940s the same kinds of expectations were once again raised by the incredible success story tied to the so-called *Army Specialized Training Program*—a method designed specifically for army personnel during World War II, so that they could learn the foreign languages they would encounter in the course of their wartime duties as quickly as possible. Based on principles of *behaviorist psychology*—which stressed habit formation and imitation—the Army Method employed two teachers. First, there was a native speaker of the language taught the new dialogue and conducted repetition exercises and pattern practice drills. During this phase, the students were given many opportunities to grasp the new material through imitation and repetition. The native speaker used only the SL. He/she introduced new vocabulary and grammatical information through oral illustrations, pictures, charts, tapes, discs, and film strips. Then, a linguist came into the classroom to provide explanations of the new grammar in the NL. This was followed by review exercises. The learning outcomes were so impressive that the Army Program was introduced into regular classrooms right after the war. However, in the schools it was found to be less successful. The reasons for this were fairly obvious to all. The classes were larger; the motivation on the part of the learners was not the same or as urgent; and only one teacher—not two (a native speaker and a linguist)—was hired to do all the instruction.

Nevertheless, the Army Program constituted a prototype for the creation of a new method that came to be known as the *Audiolingual Method* (ALM). By the early 1950s, the ALM was heralded as the "method to end all methods," i.e. as the "solution" to the SLT Dilemma for which teachers had been searching since the demise of the DM. However, in retrospect, most of the ALM's techniques were hardly new or radical. Like the DM, the ALM derived its insights from inductivist principles of learning. Its novelty lay primarily in giving these principles a new behaviorist twist:

- It stressed imitation, repetition, drills, and other kinds of habit-formation techniques.
- It emphasized the development of the four skills in chronological order—*listening-speaking-reading-writing.*
- It insisted on the formation of proper pronunciation habits from the very outset. It even used "nonsense words" to make sure that this goal was met (these were made-up forms that resembled SL words highlighting some aspect of pronunciation).
- Like the Army Program, it stressed the use of the target language for everything except explanations of grammar.
- It introduced the "language laboratory" into SLT. This allowed students to listen to prerecorded tapes and respond to cues. In this way they could assess their pronunciation and compare their efforts to those of native speakers.

The congeners of the ALM rejected the SLA = NLA hypothesis. Like Henry Sweet before them, they saw the NL as a factor that simply could not be ignored because it largely determined the ways in which students perceived and assimilated the SL. As the linguist Charles Fries (1927, 1945) observed, the motivation for this new view of SLA—known as *transfer theory*—grew out of the common observations of the errors students typically made, along with the predictable difficulties they experienced, especially during the early learning stages. Transfer theory led to the development of a new analytical technique called *contrastive analysis* (CA), which audiolingual methodologists used as the basis for designing textbooks and organizing the teaching syllabus. By "contrasting" the target and native languages, they identified which features of pronunciation, grammar, and vocabulary would require more emphasis and which ones would not. Those SL features that were identical or similar to corresponding NL ones would receive less pedagogical emphasis because the transfer process—known as *positive transfer*—would allow the students to acquire them automatically. Those that differed radically would instead receive much more instructional salience because the transfer process—known as *negative transfer*—would interfere with the student's efforts to learn the new habits and categories. In this way, positive transfer could be maximized and negative transfer minimized through pedagogical means. Those SL features and structures that were analyzed as identical or similar to the student's NL would be taught at the start of a course of study, while those that were identified as dissimilar would be taught later on.

The European counterpart to the ALM was the *Audiovisual Method* (AVM), which was developed in the 1950s in France at the *Centre du recherche et d'étude pour la diffusion du français*. The AVM was very similar in overall design to its American counterpart, stressing pattern practice, habit formation, and the teaching of oral skills before reading and writing skills. But it added an innovative feature to its basic behaviorist blueprint—the new dialogical and conversational material was introduced visually via filmstrips and other kinds of visual aids.

Teachers adopted audiolingual pedagogy *en masse* in America and Europe. However, over the years, the expectations that teachers had of the ALM were never fully met. By the mid-1960s disenchantment with audiolingualism became widespread. There were, in my view, two main reasons for this. First, like the DM, the ALM assumed that *all students* learned in essentially the *same way*. And this is simply not the case. Second, the insights of Fries and his student Robert Lado (1957, 1964) on the need to incorporate cultural patterns into a course of study were largely ignored by audiolingual textbook authors and syllabus designers. If we teach Spanish language forms but refer to American cultural meanings, values, and patterns of behavior, we are not fully teaching Spanish, but rather English thoughts clothed in Spanish words (Lado 1964: 149-150). Thus, a conversation at cross-purposes may continue indefinitely until it becomes blatantly obvious that something has gone awry. These two reasons, and not its behaviorist orientation, were behind audiolingualism's demise. Many of its innovative ideas and techniques, such as transfer theory and CA, continue to be useful as pedagogical constructs or techniques to this day, whether it is admitted or not. This is because they were born of the classroom observations of teachers, not of the intellectual ruminations of researchers.

The Cognitive-Code Method

By the mid-1960s the psychological and linguistic *Zeitgeist* had changed drastically. Behaviorism gave way to *cognitivism* in mainstream psychology (Ausubel 1967) and structuralism, on which transfer theory and CA were based, yielded to *generativism* in mainstream linguistics (Chomsky 1957, 1965). A series of psycholinguistic experiments showed, moreover, that no significant differences in oral proficiency were produced by the ALM when compared to deductivist approaches such as the GTM (e.g. Scherer and Wertheimer 1964).

Based in large part on the theoretical notions of generative linguistics, a new deductivist method emerged from the ashes of the ALM in the early 1970s. It was called the *Cognitive-Code Method* (Jakobovits 1971, Chastain 1971, Lugton 1971). At first, it seemed to provide constructive answers to the questions that teachers had raised about the ALM—e.g. Should grammar be taught explicitly before introducing dialogues and getting students to engage in structured conversations? If so, what scientific theory of grammar is the most appropriate one? The Cognitive-Code Method adopted generativist grammatical theory. It was thus formatted to impart, above all else, knowledge of abstract rules of syntax. Students were then required to apply this knowledge to meaningful tasks—such as the programming of real-life conversations. However, the Cognitive-Code Method never really caught on with teachers at large. By the mid-1970s it disappeared from the pedagogical radar screen, figuratively speaking.

However, it left behind two things of lasting value for SLT generally: (1) contextualized grammar training, and (2) the technique of Error Analysis (EA). The contextualization of grammar rules—i.e. the exemplification of how rules undergird discourse—continues to be important because it impresses upon students that syntactic structures are not mere abstractions, but rather, components of real-life conversations. Cognitive theorists distinguished *errors* from *mistakes*. They defined the latter as the blunders that students make, but which they can easily correct themselves; they defined the former, instead, as predictable and explainable deviations caused by gaps in linguistic competence. EA led shortly thereafter to *interlanguage theory*—the view that student discourse is characterized above all else by predictable, recurring errors (Selinker 1972, Richards 1974, Ludwig 1979, Corder 1981, Robinett and Schachter 1983).

EAs of student interlanguages have made it obvious that there are two general types of errors committed typically by learners: (1) *interlinguistic*, which are caused by negative transfer; and (2) *intralinguistic*, which are caused by the same general learning mechanisms that characterize NLA, i.e. by generalization, analogy, simplification, etc. An example of a typical interlinguistic error committed by English-speaking students of Italian is: **Io aspetto per Maria* = "I am waiting for Mary." The correct form is *Io aspetto Maria*. The source of this error is the negative transfer of English *for* to the formation of the Italian sentence. In Italian the verb *aspettare* is transitive, whereas in English *to wait* is intransitive (requiring the preposition *for* before the object):

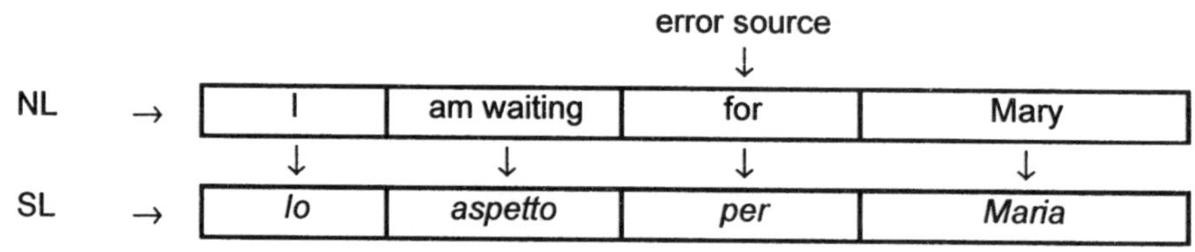

Figure 1. Negative Transfer

Intralinguistic errors are caused by general processes intrinsic to language acquisition in general. They are very similar to the developmental errors that children manifest as they speak their NL. Thus, for instance, when a non-native student of English produces the form **goed* (for *went*), he/she is guessing intelligently on the basis of what he/she knows about past-tense morphology (*play* = *played, try* = *tried,* etc.). Similarly, when a non-native student of Italian pluralizes *problema* ("problem") as *probleme* (rather than *problemi*), he/she is guessing that the rule *nouns ending in -a are pluralized by changing the -a to -e* applies to *problema*, which of course it does not.

Post-Method Responses

By the mid-1970s, interest in converting psychological and linguistic theories into pedagogical practices had waned considerably. Teachers started perceiving the dependence on these disciplines as counterproductive, because of their inbuilt instability. And, in truth, if anything has marked the histories of psychology and linguistics, it is a proclivity for theoretical partisanship, internal bickering, and a constant need to discard, rather than build upon, previous theoretical positions (behavioral theory vs. cognitive theory, structuralism vs. generativism, etc.). Moreover, teachers started questioning the implicit goal of all the methods—the development of *linguistic competence.* Rarely, they emphasized, could students use their new "competence" to do things with the SL in the real world: e.g. how to be polite, how to make social contact, how to express oneself in specific situations, etc. Imparting this kind of know-how was not considered by any of the methods (with the exception perhaps of the Oral Method) to be their primary objective, even though such *savoir-faire* was precisely what the students needed to carry out meaningful conversations with native speakers. A new view of the SLA/SLT interface had clearly emerged. By the early 1970s that view was bolstered by a new focus on *communication* in linguistics itself.

Communicative Language Teaching

It was the linguist Dell Hymes (1972) who indirectly brought about the end of the "method notion" when he argued convincingly that language systems were hardly impervious to influences from real-world social interaction. He suggested that, on the contrary, verbal structures were shaped, and over time even modified, by language use. Moreover, he argued that the ability to apply language to specific situations in a meaningful way constituted a different kind of competence. He called it *communicative competence.* Hymes' term held an instant appeal to teachers, who at the time were also beginning to suspect that the method notion was a fundamentally flawed one. The work on communicative competence in linguistics led, in turn, to a true "paradigm shift" in language education—as the philosopher Thomas Kuhn (1970) called a radical change in scientific theorizing—a shift away from the development of *linguistic competence* to a focus on *communicative competence.* This shift led to the *Communicative Language Teaching Movement.*

The first steps to develop *communicative syllabi* were taken by the Council of Europe. By the mid-1970s two highly influential syllabi, called the *Threshold Level* (Van Ek 1975) and the *Notional-Functional Syllabus* (Wilkins 1976), became widely discussed and implemented in SLT generally. The organizing principle in both was the concept of *speech act*, defined as a communicative strategy that native speakers employ unconsciously to carry out specific types of social functions. A simple protocol such as saying *hello* or *good-bye*, for instance, constitutes a "speech act" because it is based on an implicit "script" that is not unlike what occurs on a stage—i.e. it requires a detailed knowledge of the appropriate words, phrases, structures, and nonverbal cues that come together cohesively in a script-like fashion to enable a speaker to carry out a successful interaction with another speaker. An infringement of any of the procedural details of this script might lead to a breakdown in communication, confrontation, or social inappropriateness. Consider, as a case-in-point, the following common scenario in which an adolescent high school student says good-bye, first to his English teacher, second to his mother, and third to a peer:

Good-bye to English Teacher:	Good-bye, sir!
Good-bye to Mother:	See ya' later, ma!
Good-bye to a Peer:	I gotta' split, man!

Clearly, these are not interchangeable utterances—i.e. the adolescent would not say "I gotta split, man!" to a teacher, and vice versa, he would not say, "Good-bye, sir!" to a peer, because they would result as socially inappropriate and, thus, ridiculous. This simple, yet instructive, example shows that the choice of language forms and the types of structural patterns that are utilized in specific situations will vary predictably. This kind of practical knowledge is clearly part of communicative competence. The "act" of saying good-bye must be carried out by interrelating language choices with communicative situation. Drawing upon the ideas of socially-minded linguists such as Firth (1957) and Halliday (1973, 1975) and philosophers such as Austin (1962) and Searle (1969), the early architects of communicative syllabi tailored the structural information pertaining to SL grammar and vocabulary in their syllabi to reflect its uses in speech situations.

Humanistic and Neurolinguistic Methods

But not all teachers agreed with the new focus on communication in general methodology. Some started looking elsewhere for insights, reviving in the process the idea of *one method for all.* Two general trends emerged from this divergent view of SLT. The first, generally known as the *Humanistic Language Teaching Movement,* claimed that, ultimately, it was the students' emotions and personality which determined the outcome of the whole process and, thus, had to be taken directly into account; the second, known as the *Neurolinguistic Teaching Movement*, stressed that knowledge of how the brain acquired and stored information was the key towards designing an effective teaching method. Both movements were, in effect, motivated by the conviction, expressed almost sixty years earlier by Palmer, that the personality characteristics and emotional needs of the students were of paramount importance in guaranteeing successful SLA. The most widely-discussed (more so than widely-used) of these methods were as follows: Curran's *Community Counseling* (1976), Gattegno's *Silent Way* (1976), Asher's *Total Physical Response* (1977, 1981), Lozanov's *Suggestopedia* (1979), Krashen and Terrell's *Natural Approach* (1983), and Di Pietro's *Scenario Approach* (1987). Despite considerable differences in pedagogical detail, all these shared two central beliefs: (1) the need to provide a non-threatening and congenial learning environment; and (2) the need to get students involved directly in the learning process. The founders of these methods consistently reported positive results. If true, the reason for their success, however, does not require reference to any sophisticated theoretical framework—a learner who feels comfortable and a contributing participant in the learning process is bound to acquire skills more easily.

The *Neurolinguistic Methods* (NLMs) will be discussed in more detail in the next chapter. Suffice it to say here that together with the Humanistic Methods they have been pivotal in pointing out the importance of taking the student's emotional needs into direct account in SLT. The main "tenets" of their teaching philosophy can be summarized as follows:

- An obstacle to learning a language is the anxiety the learner tends to experience in the traditional language classroom. This must be removed before any learning can take place.
- The teacher needs to give students more opportunities to express themselves freely, rather than in a structured fashion.
- The students themselves should become more proactive in the whole process. They should thus be accorded more decision-making power with respect to certain aspects of syllabus design and content.
- Long-term learning is increased considerably if conditions are created in the classroom that are capable of activating unconscious processes—i.e. learning without the students realizing it.

The Proficiency Movement

The main drawback of the Humanistic Methods and of the NLMs was, and continues to be, the fact that they require the teacher's total commitment to their specific educational philosophy. For this reason, they have never really caught on with the language teaching profession at large. Moreover, by the mid-1980s general SLT practices had become much more flexible and less "trendy," as teachers sought diverse ways to resolve the SLT Dilemma. The *Proficiency Movement* in the United States, for example, led to much discussion and interesting spin-off research on how to integrate structural and communicative syllabi (Omaggio 1986, Schulz 1986). This movement stressed (and continues to emphasize) integration and *eclecticism*. Since the mid-1980s, the literature on "proficiency pedagogy" has now become an extensive one. Some the relevant insights that can be gleaned from it are central to the neuroscientific view to be discussed in the course of this book. Suffice it to say for the present purposes, that the picture emerging from the research "facts-on-file," so to speak, is that SLA, when looked at comparatively with NLA, seems to "run a certain course." But this course is not as fixed, nor as predictable, as it is in NLA. Above all else, the relevant research has shown that there are three main factors that influence the attainment of high levels of proficiency: (1) affective variables which initiate and regulate the SLA process, (2) cognitive strategies that a learner performs on the input provided to him/her in the classroom, and (3) the ability of the instructional system used to differentiate between novel and familiar learning *events*, and to reflect this difference in its *modus operandi.* Novel learning *events* are essentially characterizable as *cognizing events*, whereas the practice of already-acquired knowledge and skill is characterizable as a *recognizing event*. The key to successful SLA lies, it would seem, in determining at what point the student's *cognizing mode* is ready to become a *recognizing mode*.

As will be argued throughout this book, the former is tied primarily to the functions of the right hemisphere of the brain and can thus be called the "R-Mode," while the latter is tied primarily to the functions of the left hemisphere and can thus be labeled "L-Mode," using a terminology suggested by art instructor Betty Edwards (1979) several decades ago. As the great Russian psychologist Lev S. Vygotsky (1962) pointed out, the learner will demonstrate by his/her behavior when he/she has reached the point when the two modes become interdependent. This state will be called "intermodal" in this book. It is characterized by the ability to use cognition and recognition in tandem in the programming of language material. The attainment of intermodality will, of course, vary from student to student in terms of breadth (how much a particular individual is capable of learning something) and duration (the length of time the individual needs to grasp some learning task); but the attainment of each one will show up invariably, *for a particular student*, in appropriate linguistic behavior.

Some Issues

What the history of SLT shows, above all else, is that language teachers take their profession seriously. They simply will not give up trying to find ways that will help them make classroom SLA effective. Their attempts to resolve the SLT Dilemma in the past have provided the profession today with a catalogue of "facts-on-file" that can form the basis for developing ever-more effective approaches to the classroom. These also allow us to establish a frame-of-reference for discussing the SLA/SLT interface intelligently and constructively. The ongoing research and debate on the SLT Dilemma has, however, also produced an inventory of "unanswered issues" which, as I write, continue to form the crux of research and heated debate in the SLT profession generally. The main four issues, as I see them, are: (1) the *acquisition vs. learning* dichotomy, (2) the validity of so-called *Universal Grammar Theory*, (3) the *Critical Period Hypothesis*, and (4) the role of cultural content in syllabus design.

Acquisition vs. Learning

The distinction between *acquisition* and *learning* is due primarily to Stephen Krashen (e.g. 1985). It has great appeal because it encapsulates something that teachers have always felt intuitively—namely that students pick up certain things unconsciously, but require great conscious effort and focus to grasp other things. The former is a manifestation of *acquisition*; the latter of *learning*. Acquisition is dominant during cognizing events, when students pick up many new skills unconsciously. Learning, on the other hand, is dominant during recognizing events, when students attempt to understand "what is going on," so to speak. In NLA, acquisition governs the initial neonate period of verbal development. When infants come into contact with unfamiliar objects, their instinctive reaction is to explore them with the *senses*, i.e. to handle them, taste them, smell them, listen to any sounds they make, and visually observe their features. This exploratory phase constitutes a *sensory cognizing* stage—a stage that the Swiss psychologist Jean Piaget (1923) called appropriately the *sensory-motor stage*. During this phase infants are capable of distinguishing meaningful verbal stimuli from random noises. The mental images that result from sensory cognition allow infants to *recognize* the same objects subsequently without having, each time, to examine them over again thoroughly with their sensory apparatus. Now, as infants grow, they start to engage more and more in reflective behavior that displaces this sensory phase; i.e. they start pointing to the object and imitating the sounds it makes, rather than just handling it, tasting it, etc. These imitations and indications are the child's first attempts at *representing* the things in his/her world (Morris 1938, 1946). Piaget called this the *pre-operational stage*, since it is during this phase that children are able to operate certain tasks involving previously-formed sensory concepts. From that point on, *sensory knowing* yields to *conceptual knowing*. By the age of 7-11 years, which Piaget called the *concrete operations stage*, children become sophisticated representers of the world. At that point, they rely more and more on conscious processes to represent and know the world around them.

Krashen insists that the acquisition vs. learning dichotomy typifies classroom SLA universally. But, if this is so then: (1) When is one or the other of the modes operative? and (2) Under what conditions can or should each one be activated? According to Krashen, acquisition is the critical mode during all initial orientation tasks. For this reason, he suggests, it is crucial to ensure that the input to which students are exposed is conducive to acquisition. Learning, on the other hand, is a "secondary" mode that becomes operative when students know enough about the language to be able to reflect upon it consciously. Krashen's ideas have been debated and researched for almost two decades. Without going here into the many derivative questions and issues that the work on the acquisition vs. learning dichotomy has raised, suffice it to say that that it seems to have a fundamental "rightness" about it. In this book, acquisition will be defined as an R-Mode function and learning as an L-Mode. It is my view that both modes are required to work in tandem in the development of true proficiency. That is, in fact, the central tenet of *Bimodality Theory*—the pedagogical framework that will be developed in subsequent chapters.

Universal Grammar Theory

Within developmental psychology, there exists a considerable stockpile of research suggesting that the patterns characterizing NLA are largely predictable across cultures. This led the linguist Noam Chomsky in the 1960s to claim that human infants possess a species-specific capacity to develop their native-language grammars by simply being exposed to verbal input. The human brain, Chomsky suggested, must have a special device for detecting and reproducing language. He called it a *Language Acquisition Device* (LAD). In the 1980s, he revised his view somewhat by renaming the LAD a *Universal Grammar* (UG) (Chomsky 1986). He defined the UG as a set of innate principles of language design wired into the brain at birth that are constrained by the specific *parameters* that characterize the grammar of the particular language to which the child is exposed, so that the child can develop the *particular grammar* that his/her NL requires.

As with any overarching explanation of language, there are many problems with UG Theory. These will not be dealt with here for they are subsidiary to the main purpose at hand. In SLA circles, UG Theory has both its supporters and its opponents. One problem with the theory, as Jacobs (1988: 330) aptly puts it, is that it ignores "what the environment brings to the brain, including both the input itself (e.g. structure, intonation, morphology) and the surrounding situational variables (e.g. gestures, discourse context); and, just as importantly, must also consider what the brain does to this information." A second problem is that UG Theory assigns a unique status to the language faculty in human development. The question of whether or not it is part of a larger propensity that is also responsible for the development of musical, humor, and other nonverbal faculties is largely discarded by proponents of UG Theory.

Theoretical quibbling aside, the studies have shown that, despite considerable individual variation in the rate of the developmental process and in the order of acquisition of the specific traits of a language, children all over the world follow a similar path on the way to speech, often called *acquisition by stages* (e.g. Lenneberg 1967, Brown 1973). Among the first to document this process was the linguist Roman Jakobson (1941). Jakobson found that children learned typically to use phonemes (minimal units of distinctive sound) to refer to objects and events in their immediate environment by first distinguishing between general phonic categories (e.g. consonants vs. vowels) and then by further discriminating among the significant differences within each category—known as progressive *phonemic differentiation*. The reason for this is to be found in the neurophysiology of the brain. Phonemic distinctions are perceived by the hearing center of the brain and produced through its motor pathways via a complex neural coordination system. There are twelve cranial nerves. Seven of these link the brain with the vocal organs. Some perform a motor function, controlling the movement of muscles; while others perform a sensory function, sending signals to the brain. The larynx controls the flow of air to and from the lungs, so as to prevent food, foreign objects, or other substances from entering the trachea on their way to the stomach. The ability to control the vocal folds makes it possible to build up pressure within the lungs and to emit air not only for expiration purposes, but also for the production of sound. In order for phonemic discrimination to emerge, this neurophysiological system must develop first or in tandem with speech processes. Only then can this system serve language acquisition productively.

The research on NLA has, since Jakobson's pivotal work, established certain milestones in verbal development. These can be synthesized as follows. After an initial cooing stage that starts virtually at birth, around six months children begin babbling and eventually imitating the linguistic sounds they hear in the immediate environment. These imitations lead to the first words, which are monosyllabic reductions of adult words—*ma* for *mama*, *da* for *dog*, *ca* for *cat*, etc. These constitute the first acts of conceptual, rather than pure sensory, knowing. At eight months reduplications and imitative repetitions become more frequent in child discourse. Moreover, children start employing intonation patterns distinctly to convey emotional states. By the end of the first year, the first true words emerge (*mama, dada*, etc.). In the 1960s, the psycholinguist Martin Braine (1963, 1971) noticed that these single words gradually embodied the communicative functions of entire phrases: e.g. the child's word *dada* could mean "Where is daddy"? "I want daddy," etc. according to situation. He called them *holophrastic*, or one-word, utterances. In situations of normal upbringing, holophrases reveal that a vast amount of neurophysiological and conceptual development has taken place in the child by the end of the first year of life. During the holophrastic stage, in fact, children can name objects, express actions or the desire to carry out actions, and transmit emotional states rather effectively (Cruttenden 1974).

Holophrases are the result of imitation. But the imitation deployed is hardly pure mimicry. It is a creative form of simulation. Children imitate what they hear and then create forms on the basis of it. Over 60% of their "constructive creations" will develop into nouns, and 20% will become verbs. In a study of four infants from different language backgrounds, Boysson-Bardies and Vihman (1991) found that the actual forms and functions that holophrases take depend not only on developmental neurophysiological constraints and on the specific language input to which a child is exposed. The early holophrases are, in effect, the first products of the child's attempts to transform imitative states of knowing into conceptual ones. By 16-18 months, the child starts manifesting a remarkable ability to employ holophrastic language creatively. As Vygotsky (1961: 298) aptly put it: "The primary word is not a straightforward symbol for a concept but rather an image, a picture, a mental sketch of a short concept, a short tale about it—indeed, a small work of art."

During the second year, the child's ability to use intonation increases rapidly, reaching adult norms. The child then passes on to what Braine (1971) called the *telegraphic stage*—a stage characterized by two- and three-word utterances. He termed it *telegraphic* because, as in the composition of a telegram, children construct their utterances in a condensed fashion, without all the elements that characterize adult syntax: *More milk, Daddy home*, etc. Braine claimed that telegraphic utterances were grounded on a "pivot grammar," given that some of the words functioned as grammatical pivots (*more*, *less*, etc.) while others belonged to a more open lexical class (*milk*, *candy*, etc.). This pivot grammar seems to function as a verbal backbone around which the acquisition of vocabulary increases dramatically and rapidly. As children enter this stage, they have knowledge of about 270 words. By the age of 4-5, they can manage thousands of words.

UG Theory can, of course, account for the fact that NLA follows such distinct stages universally, no matter where a language is acquired or what that language is. To account for differences in grammatical organization, Chomsky proposed the notion of "parameters," i.e. of organizational subprinciples that allow a specific language to take shape from the fund of general principles in the brain's UG. But this apparently "accurate" explanation of the facts actually ignores two other kinds of facts that put a "fly into its theoretical ointment," so to speak. First, UG Theory cannot explain the critical role played by imitation in early NLA. Second, it ignores the role played by other abilities in childhood (drawing, music, humor, etc.), given that these develop in tandem with language and are just as species-specific as language.

In the area of SLA, UG Theory would seem to exclude the possibility of successful acquisition because of the diminishing operability of the UG (or the LAD) after puberty. It has, in fact, been used opportunely by some to explain why SLA in adolescence and adulthood is so difficult, when compared to NLA. But, again, why do some (and perhaps many) acquire an SL after puberty nonetheless? At present, the research on UG Theory within SLA has not answered any of the questions raised here in any satisfactory way. The lack of success in acquiring an SL after puberty may be due to a host of mitigating and overlapping factors that we know virtually nothing about. One of these is the relation of language to the user's native conceptual system—a topic that will be taken in up in some detail in subsequent chapters. Another is, of course, motivation. The motivation studies throughout the years have shown continually that there is a positive correlation between motivation and success at language learning.

The Critical Period Hypothesis

The reformers assumed, as we saw above, that SLA ran the same "acquisition route" as NLA. They believed that they would be able to "activate" acquisition in the classroom by designing an appropriate teaching method. In 1967, the linguist Eric Lenneberg cast serious doubt on the reformist paradigm by claiming that the *critical period* for language acquisition was from birth to about puberty. After the critical period, the brain lost its ability to acquire a new language *to the same degree* that was possible in childhood. The negative implications of Lenneberg's *Critical Period Hypothesis* (CPH) for solving the SLT Dilemma were immediately obvious to teachers of all methodological stripes. But these hardly discouraged them. On the contrary, the CPH spurred them on even more so to find a suitable way to solve the SLT Dilemma once and for all, no matter what some neurolinguists claimed.

The two questions that teachers sought to examine in the aftermath of the CPH were the following ones: (1) Was SLA truly blocked by neurology after the critical period? (2) If not, was SLA characterized by the same kinds of stages and processes that characterized NLA? Like their reformer predecessors, teachers argued *en masse* that true proficiency in the SL was possible after puberty, but that it took time, patience, and a significant effort on the part of both teacher and learner to "make it happen." Moreover, as Krashen and others emphasized, the behavior of typical students in classroom environments suggests strongly that the so-called LAD hardly stopped operating after puberty. On the contrary, it appears to be just as operative in the post-pubescent period, since many of the same unconscious processes that characterize NLA surface constantly in the observable learning behaviors of students *of all ages*. From the research on interlanguages in the 1970s, moreover, it seemed that SLA followed a "natural order," given that errors were seen as forming a sequential pattern, by which certain structures are acquired early and others later. This suggested to many that SLA was quite similar to NLA and certainly not blocked by maturational processes. *Stage models* of SLA were thus proposed, discussed, developed, and intensely researched (Obler 1980, Galloway and Krashen 1980, Krashen 1985, Gass and Madden 1985).

The CPH will be discussed in subsequent chapters. It is sufficient to note here that it may be true in part—especially with regard to the acquisition of SL pronunciation. But, like UG Theory it ignores far too much the role of context, motivation, and other factors that always enter into the learning picture—as teachers know all too well.

The Role of Culture

As the ancients knew, people seem to develop high levels of proficiency when they become immersed in the cultures of the communities that speak the language than they do by being exposed to the language in classroom settings. The reason for this is rather obvious—learning a language in its natural cultural context allows the student to interrelate its forms and uses to the broader *conceptual system* to which it is tied. Each language is designed to encode concepts in different ways. The more distant the cultural and historical relation between languages, the greater the conceptual differences between them. Although people may see the same rainbow, the number and range of the rainbow's *hues* they can name will depend on how many color terms have been encoded by the languages they speak. Some languages have everyday words for a dozen colors; others can get by with only a couple. Cultures leave uncoded those aspects of reality that they consider unimportant to them. For example, given the world they inhabit, the nomadic Canadian Inuit have had little interest in distinguishing hues for different types of plants; what they needed were words to talk about different kinds of snow. That is why in some Inuit dialects more than 50 words referring to ice and snow are still in use.

The question for SLT that this kind of discussion raises is an obvious one: How can the immersion experience be transferred to the classroom? Or, more specifically: How can SLT interrelate the new language to the conceptual system of the culture that speaks it? In the late 1970s, the Research Center for Language and Semiotic Studies at Indiana University aimed to answer this very question, under the directorship of the renowned linguist and semiotician Thomas A. Sebeok. From that project, it became obvious that one way to bring culture into the classroom, so to speak, was to tie the SL to the nonverbal aspects of its delivery in conversations. As a consequence, a handbook on nonverbal communication for teachers of Japanese was published, accompanied by a half-hour film in which native Japanese speakers were seen to execute culturally-appropriate gestures as they spoke about certain topics. That and other films made it saliently obvious to teachers how intrinsically interconnected the gestural and verbal modes are in any act of message delivery (Rector and Trinta 1985). The Indiana project subsequently inspired a series of critical studies in the 1980s examining the role of "body language" and gesture in SLA (e.g. Raffler-Engel 1980, Arndt and Pesch 1984, Poyatos 1989, Diadori 1990).

Recent research on concepts in SLA (e.g. Russo 1997) is beginning to show that learning a new language is not a simple matter of learning how to articulate new sounds and how to use new word-making patterns to communicate something. It involves, rather, learning how linguistic, nonverbal, and conceptual systems interact. Consider, as a simple case-in-point, the difference between *orologio* in Italian and *watch* and *clock* in English. The Italian and English words refer at a denotative level to "a mechanical device for registering the passage of time." But in English the two words call attention to the "portability" of the device—*watches* are worn or carried, *clocks* are put on tables, hung on walls, etc. No such attention is necessitated by the word *orologio*. The notion of "portability" is not relevant in the use of *orologio*, but that of "location" is (*table clock, wrist watch*, etc.). In Italian this is conveyed by *da* + "location": e.g. *orologio da tavolo* "table clock," *orologio da polso* "wrist watch," *orologio da muro* "wall clock," etc.

The primary reason why student discourse manifests a high degree of "conceptual unnaturalness" is, undoubtedly, the fact that rarely have students been exposed to the relation between linguistic and conceptual systems. But even simply exposing students to culture-specific concepts through reading texts, visual materials, realia, etc. is not sufficient. Rather, it will be necessary to develop a pedagogical approach that interrelates the new language and the culture-specific conceptual system it reflects in a direct fashion. That will be the target of discussion of the fourth chapter of this book.

The Foray into the Neurosciences

The NLMs (Neurolinguistic Methods) mentioned briefly above constitute the first practical attempts to tackle the SLT Dilemma by taking the "source" of all learning—the brain—directly into account. The congeners of those methods saw SLA as a process involving *neurological reorganization*. So, they each devised a pedagogical system that, they claimed, would bring this reorganization about. However, as we shall see in the next chapter, the NLMs stumbled into the same trap in which the DM fell by assuming that *all students* learned in the same way. Nevertheless, their foray into the neuroscientific domain has been a very important one for SLT in general, leading to a host of ideas about what to do to make classroom SLA more "brain-compatible."

The human brain is a grayish-pink, jelly-like ball with many ridges and grooves on its surface. A newborn's brain weighs less than 1 pound (0.5 kilograms). By the time the infant reaches 6 years of age, the brain has reached its full weight of about 3 pounds (1.4 kilograms). It is the master control center of the body, constantly receiving information from the senses about conditions both inside and outside the body. It rapidly analyzes this information and then sends out messages that control body functions and actions. The brain also stores information from past experience, which makes learning and remembering possible. It is the source of thoughts, moods, and emotions. Clearly, knowledge of how this organ works and what can be done to make it work *efficiently* in artificial situations, such as classrooms, is vital knowledge that has concrete implications for designing methodology, textbooks, syllabi, learning materials, etc.

In neuroscientific discussions of SLT, various terms are used, at times interchangeably and at others distinctively. The main ones are as follows:

- *Neurology:* is the branch of medicine that studies the nervous system and its diseases.
- *Neurophysiology:* is the branch of biology and neuroscience that studies how nerve cells, called neurons, receive and transmit information.
- *Neuroscience:* is the science that studies all aspects of the relation between brain and mind.
- *Neuropsychology:* is the branch of neuroscience that studies how brain processes undergird psychological processes.
- *Neurolinguistics:* is the branch of neuroscience that studies the various aspects of the relation between the brain and language.

Neuroscientists have been putting together a rather substantive profile of how language is organized in the brain. Some evidence has emerged, for instance, that bilinguals and advanced SL learners are equally lateralized in each of their languages; that there might be a greater right hemisphere involvement in the early stages of SLA; and so on. However, I should alert the reader to the fact that in their enthusiasm, neuroscientifically-inclined researchers and teachers have perhaps not always been judicious and cautious in applying brain theories and notions to SLT pedagogy. I cannot but agree with Spolsky (1989: 86) when he remarked a while back that "the body of hard data on the neuroscience of second language learning comes nowhere near matching the enormous amount of speculation or the large number of studies." Nevertheless, if any true progress is to be made in solving the SLT Dilemma, I firmly believe that the path to pursue is the one laid out by the NLMs. In my view, the more the teacher is familiar with the brain research, the more he/she will be able to respond appropriately to the various situations that present themselves in the classroom.

The critical pattern that those methods have uncovered is that there is a "flow" that seems to characterize most types of novel learning tasks in SLA. Consequently, determining which learning tasks are novel and which ones are not is the critical point-of-departure for developing any instructional game plan. Discussing the pedagogical implications of this "neuroscientific principle" is one of the main goals of the remainder of this book. In a sense, it is a modern-day reformulation of what is actually the oldest principle in education—the *inductivist principle*. According to this principle, the conditions that foster true proficiency are those that involve a flow from experiential to expository learning, from practical to theoretical content, and from concrete to analytical instruction for novel learning tasks.

The reformer's theory-into-practice paradigm was so full of promise that it conditioned teachers throughout the twentieth century to wait for "experts" to hand them down a pedagogical system that would allow them to make classroom language learning effortless and bring about high levels of proficiency. The paradigm also predisposed them to think that any "fault" in a given pedagogical proposal would subsequently be eliminated as psychologists gained more knowledge about human learning and linguists about the nature of language. This led to a tendency to overhaul previous pedagogy any time the theoretical coordinates in psychology and linguistics shifted—a proclivity that constantly interrupted the development of a coherent strategy for tackling the SLT Dilemma. As we saw, the "hand-me-down" syndrome was greatly tempered in the 1970s, when more and more teachers started to realize that psychology and linguistics did not have all the answers. If there were any "answers" to be gleaned from a theoretical domain, then it would have to be the teachers themselves who found them, not the theorists which, incidentally, is exactly what the reformers had in mind in the first place.

CHAPTER 2
LOOKING TO BRAIN RESEARCH FOR INSIGHTS

I consider that a man's brain originally is like a little empty attic, and you have to stock it with such furniture as you choose.

Sir Arthur Conan Doyle (1859-1930)

Introduction

As mentioned in the previous chapter, Eric Lenneberg's watershed 1967 study on the *Biological Foundations of Language* seemed, at first, to give a fatal blow to the hopes that the reformist paradigm had raised up till then, for the simple reason that it appeared to negate the possibility of SLA after the age of puberty. Lenneberg called the period before puberty the *critical* one for language acquisition. He developed this notion after reviewing an extensive corpus of aphasiology data—data on individuals who had suffered language impairments, called *aphasias*, caused by damage to specific language areas in their brains. From his review, Lenneberg noted a pattern. It was statistically more likely for those who incurred left hemisphere brain damage before puberty to have their native language taken over by the right hemisphere. In effect, most aphasics developed language before puberty, despite their early impairments. However, after puberty Lenneberg noted that aphasias tended to become permanent. By extrapolation, he concluded that in normal individuals the ability to acquire a new language after puberty diminished considerably. This had obvious negative implications for SLT. Simply put, if Lenneberg's CPH (Critical Period Hypothesis) were in fact true, then it would be a waste of time to continue tackling the SLT Dilemma through pedagogical means.

Shortly after Lenneberg's book came out, and gained widespread renown, SL teachers reacted swiftly and critically. Some suspected that Lenneberg had interpreted the aphasiology data in a biased manner, so as to lend support to the Chomskyan innatist view of language. They argued that factors other than biological ones were at work in language acquisition at all periods of life. Others decided to ignore the CPH completely, looking at the relevant brain research from an entirely different perspective—to extract insights that would purportedly help them solve the SLT Dilemma once and for all.

The latter reaction has, in my view, been the most productive one for SLT. Since the early 1970s, in fact, interest among SL educators in the brain sciences has increased considerably. The questions that this "neuroscientific trend" has raised generally for the study SLA, and the practical insights it has produced for SLT, will be discussed in this chapter. But before doing so, it is essential to provide a schematic outline of relevant brain physiology, as well as a brief historical survey of neuroscience, in order to establish a background to the discussion to follow in this and subsequent chapters.

The Brain

Knowing about basic brain functions and being able to name the various parts of the brain has no direct implications for SLT. Nevertheless, it is useful to have this kind of knowledge for two practical reasons: (1) the SLA literature has been employing neuroscientific terms and concepts increasingly since the early 1970s, and (2) all neuroscientific models and theories of SLT, such as the ones to be discussed in this book, utilize neuroscientific ideas to varying degrees. In a phrase, knowledge of the brain is fast becoming part of the "shop talk" that researchers and practitioners use to discuss SLA and SLT professionally.

The brain has three main sections: (1) the *cerebrum*, (2) the *cerebellum*, and (3) the *brain stem*. Each one consists chiefly of nerve cells, called *neurons*, and supporting cells, called *glia*. The hard, thick bones of the skull shield the brain from blows that could otherwise seriously injure it. In addition, three protective membranes, called *meninges,* cover the brain. The outermost membrane is the tough *dura mater*, which lines the inner surface of the skull. A thinner membrane, the *arachnoid*, lies just beneath the dura mater. The delicate *pia mater* directly covers the brain. It follows the folds of the brain's surface and contains blood vessels that carry blood to and from the cerebral cortex. A clear liquid, called *cerebrospinal fluid*, separates the pia mater and the arachnoid. This fluid forms a thin cushioning layer between the soft tissues of the brain and the hard bones of the skull.

The blood-brain barrier safeguards brain tissues from any damage that could result from contact with certain large molecules carried in the bloodstream. Substances in the blood reach body tissues by passing through the thin walls of tiny blood vessels called *capillaries.* Much of this flow occurs through the spaces between the cells that make up the capillary walls. The cells in brain capillaries are more tightly packed than they are in other capillaries, allowing them to restrict the passage of substances from the blood to the brain. The brain needs large molecules for nutrition, however. For this reason, the capillary walls have certain enzymes and other properties that enable such molecules to pass through.

Some reflex actions do not involve the brain. If someone touches a hot cup of coffee, for instance, pain impulses flash to that person's spinal cord, which immediately sends back a message to withdraw the hand. But the brain does play various roles in coordinating most other kinds of movements. For example, the *basal ganglia*, which are groups of brain cells that lie at the base of the cerebrum, help control habitualized movement sequences involved in such activities as walking and eating.

Individual brains can differ significantly, depending not only on genetics, but also on life experiences. The fingers activate the same general area of the cortex in everyone's brain. But this area is larger in people who use their fingers particularly often—for example, people who play musical instruments such as the piano or the violin, or people who read Braille (an alphabet of small raised dots developed for the blind). Neuroscientists have also found evidence that the brains of men and women differ. The *corpus callosum*—the thick band of nerve fibers connecting the cerebral hemispheres—is larger in women than it is in men. Careful examinations of brains after death have also shown that women have about 10 percent more neurons in the cortex than men. What such differences entail psychologically is not clear. In my view, culture and life experiences have more to do with psychological differences than does brain physiology.

The Cerebrum and the Cerebellum

The cerebrum makes up about 85 percent of the brain's weight. A large groove called the *longitudinal fissure* divides it into halves called the *left (cerebral) hemisphere* (LH) and the *right (cerebral) hemisphere* (RH). The hemispheres are connected by bundles of nerve fibers, the largest of which is the *corpus callosum.* Four *lobes* (regions) make up each hemisphere—each having the same name as the bone of the skull that lies above it. The lobes are: (1) the *frontal lobe* at the front; (2) the *temporal lobe* at the lower side; (3) the *parietal lobe* in the middle; and (4) the *occipital lobe* at the rear. Fissures in the cerebral cortex form the boundaries between the lobes. The two major fissures are the *central fissure* and the *lateral fissure.* Impulses from the eyes travel to the visual cortex in the occipital lobes. Portions of the temporal lobes receive messages from the ears. The area for taste lies buried in the lateral fissure, and the center of smell is on the underside of the frontal lobes.

A thin layer of nerve cell bodies makes up the *cerebral cortex*, which forms the outermost part of the cerebrum. It is also called the *neocortex*, since in evolutionary terms it is a later development than other brain structures. Most of the cerebrum beneath the cortex consists of nerve cell fibers. Some of these connect parts of the cortex; others link the cortex with the cerebellum, brain stem, and spinal cord. The cortex has many ridges and grooves, greatly increasing its surface area and the number of neurons it contains within the limited space of the skull. There is a *somatosensory* region in the cortex that receives messages from the sense organs as well as touch and temperature messages from the entire body. It lies in the parietal lobe of each hemisphere along the central fissure. Areas in the frontal lobes comprise a *motor* region. This sends out nerve impulses that control the voluntary movements of all the skeletal muscles. The motor cortex of the LH controls movements on the right side of the body, while the motor cortex of the RH directs movements on the left side of the body. More than 90 percent of human beings are right-handed because the left motor cortex, which directs the right hand, is dominant over the right motor cortex, which directs the left hand. The largest portion of the cortex is called the *association cortex.* This is involved in the analysis, processing, and storage of information, thus making possible all our higher mental abilities, such as thinking, speaking, and remembering. Below is a "map" of the cortex:

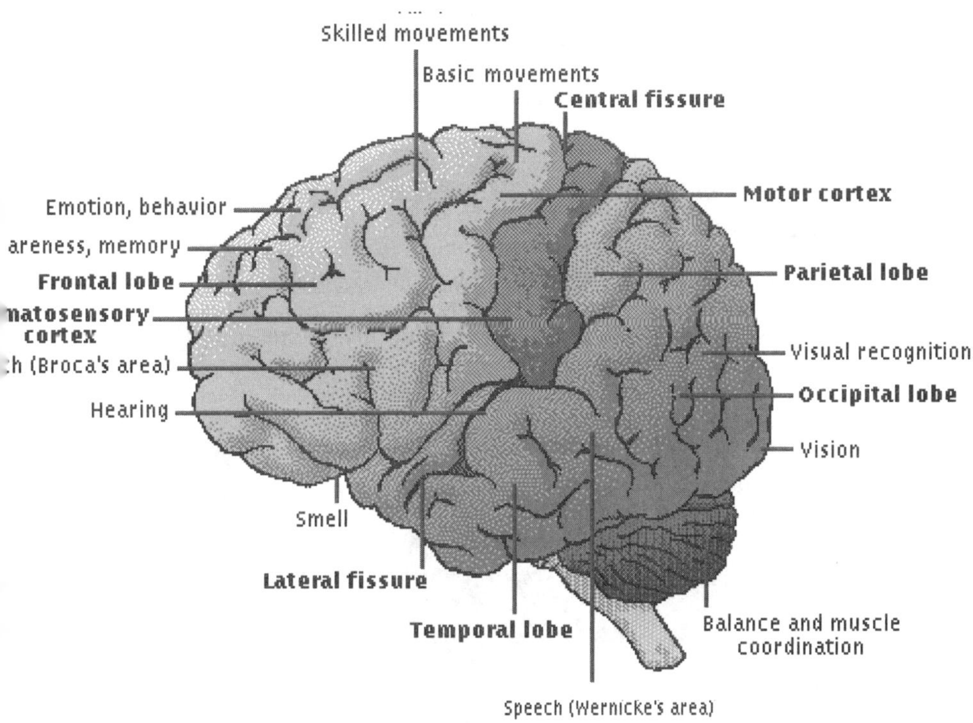

Figure 2. The Human Cortex

The cerebellum lies below the back part of the cerebrum. It consists of a large mass of closely packed *folia* (leaf-like bundles of nerve cells) which coordinate the muscle movements regulated by the motor cortex. Nerve impulses alert the cerebellum when the motor cortex "orders" a part of the body to perform a certain action. Almost instantly, impulses from that part of the body inform the cerebellum how the action is being carried out. It then compares the actual movement with the intended movement, signaling the motor cortex to make any necessary corrections or adjustments. In this way, the cerebellum ensures that the body moves smoothly and efficiently.

The cerebral cortex and the cerebellum together largely regulate voluntary movements. The motor cortex in each cerebral hemisphere sends nerve impulses to the particular muscles used in an activity, such as writing or throwing a ball. The largest areas of the motor cortex control those parts of the body that make the most complicated and precise movements. One of these controls the lips and tongue. Much smaller areas control the relatively simple movements made by such parts as the back and shoulders.

The two hemispheres are separated by a finger-shaped structure called the *vermis*. The surface of each hemisphere consists of convolutions of tissue that increase the cortical surface area available within the confines of the skull. The hemispheres are designed to share the "mental labor" of human cognition in a patterned fashion. Essentially, the RH is the seat of synthetic, imaginative, and spatial thinking; the LH of analytical, reflective, and verbal thinking. The following diagram shows how the major functions are distributed according to hemisphere:

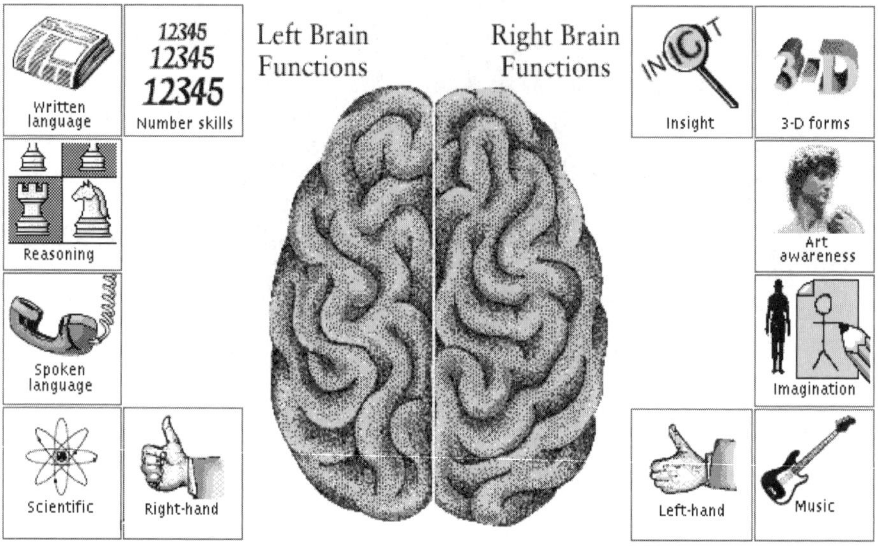

Figure 3. Functions according to Hemisphere

Speech is controlled by three main areas of the LH: (1) *Broca's area* lying just beneath the motor cortex, which is responsible for the muscle movements of the throat and mouth used in speaking; (2) *Wernicke's area*, between the auditory and visual areas, which controls comprehension; and (3) a "supplementary area" discovered by the Canadian neurologist Wilder Penfield and his associates in the 1950s (e.g. Penfield and Rasmussen 1950, Penfield and Roberts 1959), which is involved in several functions previously thought to be restricted to Broca's and Wernicke's areas.

The Brain Stem

The brain stem is a stalk-like structure that connects the cerebrum with the spinal cord. The bottom part of the brain stem is called the *medulla oblongata.* It has nerve centers that control breathing, the heartbeat, and many other vital body processes. Just above it is the *pons*, which connects the hemispheres. The pons also contains nerve fibers that link the cerebellum and the cerebrum. Above the pons lies the *midbrain*. Nerve centers in the midbrain help control movements of the eyes and the size of the pupils. At the upper end of the brain stem are the *hypothalamus* and the *thalamus.* There are actually two *thalami*, one on the left side of the brain stem and one on the right side. Each one receives nerve impulses from various parts of the body and routes them to the appropriate areas of the cerebral cortex. The thalami also relay impulses from one part of the brain to another. The hypothalamus regulates body temperature, hunger, and other internal states and conditions. It also controls the activities of the nearby *pituitary* gland, the master gland of the body. A slender stalk of tissue connects the hypothalamus with the pituitary. The hypothalamus indirectly regulates many body processes by controlling the pituitary's production and release of chemical messengers called *hormones*. Among other functions, these regulate the body's rate of growth and its sexual and reproductive processes.

The main control centers for body processes are in the brain stem. Nerve centers in the medulla regulate such functions as breathing, heartbeat, and blood flow. Other areas within the brain stem control swallowing and the movements of the stomach and intestines. The hypothalamus also has nerve centers that control processes that maintain constant conditions within the body. For example, some centers regulate the amount of water in the body. Certain nerve cells detect changes in the level of water in the body's blood and tissues and relay this information to the hypothalamus. If the water level is too low, the hypothalamus produces the sensation of thirst, which causes the person to drink water. At the same time, the hypothalamus sends messages that cause the kidneys to reduce the amount of water they remove from the body. If the water level becomes too high, the messages from the hypothalamus eliminate thirst and increase the amount of water removed by the kidneys. Other centers in the hypothalamus operate on the same principle in regulating hunger and body temperature.

A network of nerve fibers called the *reticular formation* lies deep within the brain stem. This helps regulate and maintain the brain's level of awareness. Sensory messages that pass through the brain stem stimulate the reticular formation, which in turn stimulates alertness and activity throughout the cerebral cortex.

Neuronal Structure

The human brain is essentially one huge "cellular organ." It has from 10 billion to 100 billion cells called *neurons*. All of these are formed within a few months after birth. From around 20 years of age onwards, some die off each day, without being replaced during a person's lifetime. However, this loss equals less than 10 percent of all the neurons. The neurons connect with one another in the form of complex networks. All physical and mental functioning depends on the establishment and maintenance of these networks. When a person stops performing an activity, the neural networks for the activity fall into disuse and eventually may die off.

Each neuron consists of a cell body and a number of tube-like fibers. The longest fiber, called the *axon*, carries nerve impulses from the cell body to other neurons. Short, branching fibers called *dendrites* pick up impulses from the axons of other neurons and transmit them to the cell body. The area where a branch of one neuron transmits a nerve impulse to a branch of another neuron is called a *synapse*. Each neuron may form synapses with thousands of other nerve cells:

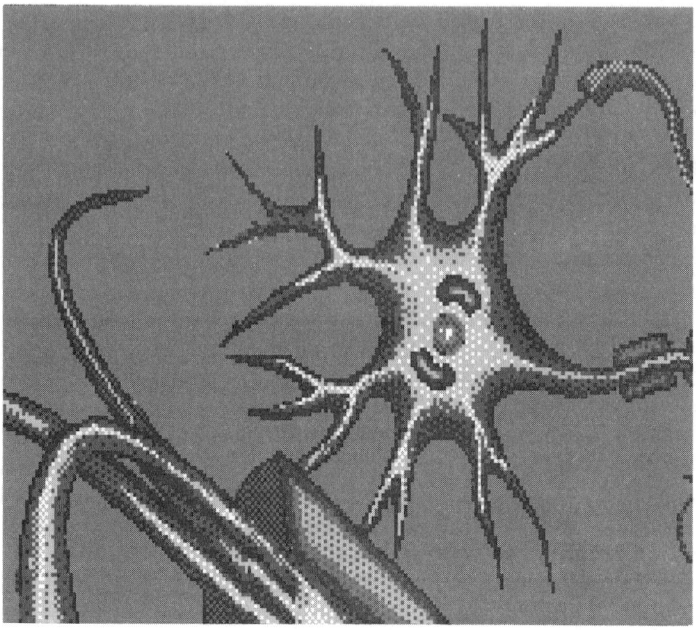

Figure 4. Synapse

Some axons have a coating of a white fatty material called *myelin*, which insulates the cell's fiber and speeds the transmission of impulses along its surface. Myelin and tightly packed axons form the so-called *white matter*. The cell bodies of neurons and the axons without myelin sheaths make up the *gray matter* of the brain. Neurons are surrounded by *glia*. These are cells that provide a supportive framework for the neurons. Glia carry out many other important tasks. For example, certain glia keep the brain free of injured and diseased neurons by engulfing and digesting them. Other glia produce the myelin sheaths that insulate some axons. Research using cells grown in laboratories also indicates that glia, like neurons, may transmit some nerve impulses.

A nerve impulse is an electro-chemical process controlled by the neuronal membrane. The latter, which has pores, maintains varying concentrations of ions inside the neuron and in its surrounding fluids. *Ions* are electrically charged atoms. As the membrane selectively allows ions to enter and leave the cell, an electric charge—the nerve impulse—travels along the neuron. Certain chemicals called *neurotransmitters* make it possible for a nerve impulse to travel from the axon of one neuron to the dendrite of another. An impulse cannot be transmitted electrically across the *synaptic cleft*, the tiny gap between the axon and the dendrite. Instead, when an impulse reaches the end of the axon, it triggers the release of neurotransmitter molecules from the cell. These cross the synaptic cleft and attach themselves to sites called *receptors* on the dendrite of the other neuron. This action alters the electrical activity of the receiving neuron in one of two ways: (1) some transmitters stimulate the neuron to produce a nerve impulse; (2) others instead prevent the neuron from producing an impulse. Neurons may manufacture more than one neurotransmitter, and their membrane surfaces may contain receptors for more than a single transmitter. A neuron also has the capacity to "learn" from past experience and change the proportions of its various neurotransmitters and receptors.

All the brain's functions depend on the normal action of neurotransmitters. An excess or deficiency of a specific transmitter or group of transmitters may lead to a serious disorder in thought, mood, or behavior.

Memory

Neuroscientists have only an elementary understanding of the extraordinarily complicated processes involved in remembering. *Memory* can be defined neurologically as the formation of neuronal circuits designed to interpret new incoming stimuli in terms of their structure as *new* or *familiar*. It has been found that certain structures of the limbic system also play major roles in this interpretive process, such as the *amygdaloid complex* and the *hippocampus*, both in the temporal lobe. Individuals who suffer damage to these structures tend to lose the ability to form new memories, even though they may retain information about events occurring before the damage. These individuals can learn new physical skills, but when performing them do not remember having done the activities before.

Whereas learning something new involves *cognition*, memorizing is an act of *recognition* (chapter 1). Cognition entails the formation of neuronal circuits; recognition of their utilization to assess the incoming information as new or familiar. Recognition also comprises the ability of neuronal circuits to reconstruct information on the basis of partial cues. Known as *recollection*, this form of memory suggests that neuronal circuits are "proactive," i.e. they have the ability to "fill in the gaps," so to speak, in the form and contents of incoming stimuli. But memory circuits are also "retroactive," allowing individuals to reacquire familiar information that has been lost over time through relearning (i.e. through the reconstruction of synaptic circuitry).

Some neuroscientists suggest that memories are stored at specific sites; but many others argue that they involve widespread brain regions working together. Both processes may in fact be involved. Specific areas seem to be involved in *short-term* (temporary) memory, whereas various neuronal networks throughout the brain are involved instead in *long-term* (permanent) memory. Either process brings about changes at the synapses—i.e. in the regions where impulses pass from one neuron to another. These may be controlled by glycoproteins or other large molecules. Extensive research will be required to verify this general explanation of memory formation and to unravel the specific details of the processes involved.

Historical Background

It was the Hippocratic physicians around 400 BC who developed the first scientific notions of brain structure in the Western world. The Greek physician Galen (c. 130-c. 200 AD) subsequently claimed that the brain was the primary organ for all human sensations and emotions and that it carried out its functions in specific ways. The first true attempts to develop a classification system for assigning mental functions to specific cerebral sites, however, had to await the fifteenth century and sixteenth centuries. Unfortunately, most of those attempts were based on speculation rather than on empirical evidence. It was believed, for instance, that the functions were localized in different ventricles—the internal cavities of brain tissue. Three centuries later, the German physician Johann Gesner studied brain functions in a more empirical fashion, arguing that deficiencies in certain behaviors were caused by a lack of communication between certain parts of the brain. Shortly thereafter, however, the German scientist Franz Joseph Gall (1758-1828) began classifying the brain once again in a speculative manner. Gall posited, for instance, that certain traits such as memory and love depended on brain size. The reaction against Gall's classification method, known as *phrenology*, was quick and effectual. Leading the charge were prominent scientists such as Jean-Baptiste Bouillaud (1796-1881), Gustave Fritsch (1838-1927), and Edouard Hitzig (1838-1907), who argued that more reliable clinical evidence was required for localizing functions in a scientifically-plausible way.

Such evidence came forth in 1861. That was the year in which the French anthropologist and neurologist Pierre-Paul Broca (1824-1880) published a paper linking a specific area in the left hemisphere of the brain to aphasia. Broca noticed a destructive lesion in the left frontal lobe during the autopsy of a patient who had lost the ability to articulate words during his lifetime, even though he had not suffered any paralysis of his speech organs. Broca concluded that the capacity to articulate speech was thus traceable to that specific cerebral site—which shortly thereafter came to bear his name (*Broca's area*). That was the watershed discovery that established, once and for all, a direct link between a mental capacity and a specific area of the brain. For the sake of historical accuracy, it should be mentioned that the military surgeon Marc Dax had presented similar evidence in 1836 at the Congrès Méridional de Montpellier, relating a destructive lesion in the LH to language loss. However, his paper was never published (Joanette, Goulet, and Hannequin 1990: 1-2). And in the same year of 1836, a Scottish physician named John Abercrombie published a paper in which he associated LH damage with verbal deficits (Obler and Gjerlow 1999: 27). However, it is Broca to whom history has conferred the distinction of being the first to make an empirically-based connection between an area of the brain and a cognitive function.

Broca was also the one who established that there existed an *asymmetry* between the brain and the body—a touch on the right side of the body, for example, is perceived in the left somatosensory area. The relation between handedness and language is now known to be largely asymmetrical. In the majority of right-handers (almost 99%), speech is controlled by the LH of the brain, as it is in about 70% of left-handers. However, in some left-handers, both hemispheres of the brain are capable of controlling speech. The RH is specialized instead for the recognition of faces and the perception of spatial relationships in both right- and left-handers. However, in the latter, some hemispheric variation is also possible.

Right after Broca's discovery, the study of aphasias became the basis for mapping the brain's linguistic sites. If damage to a specific cerebral site brought about a specific type of linguistic impairment, then that the site could be inferred to control the function in question in healthy brains. For instance, damage to Broca's area, which is in the left frontal lobe, impairs the ability to perform verbal actions (such as pronunciation). Broca's aphasics also have trouble with verbs, since these are stored in the same cortical neighborhood that controls actions. Damage to Wernicke's area, on the other hand, generally leads to a loss of comprehension. Wernicke's aphasics can articulate and perceive word forms easily, but they have a difficult time processing their meanings correctly. Damage to the left temporal lobe impairs the ability to find words and name objects and things—a syndrome known as *anomic aphasia* (Weisler and Milekic 2000: 298-299).

Not all verbal deficits result from brain damage. Some are caused by genetic abnormalities. One of these is the condition known as *Specific Language Impairment* (SLI). Sufferers from SLI are normal in all respects except in the fact that they manifest great difficulties in the area of morphology. They have no clue, for instance, how to pluralize nouns or conjugate verbs. Another is the condition known as *Williams Syndrome*, which was first described in 1961. This affects both body and brain, giving those who have it a strange and incongruous jumble of deficits and strengths. Williams sufferers have diminished cognitive capacities and heart problems, and age prematurely; yet they have outgoing personalities. They resemble each other noticeably, having wide-set hazel eyes, upturned noses, and wide mouths. Surprisingly, they show extraordinary knowledge of vocabulary. However, their ability to select words appropriately is impaired. A Williams sufferer may say *tiger* when *cat* is intended.

Cerebral Dominance Theory

Thirteen years after Broca's discovery, in 1874, the German neurologist Carl Wernicke (1848-1904) published further evidence linking the LH to language. Wernicke documented cases in which damage to another area of the LH consistently produced a recognizable pattern of impairment to the faculty of speech comprehension. Then, in 1892 the physiologist Jules Déjerine published findings showing that reading and writing deficits resulted primarily from damage to Broca's, Wernicke's, and surrounding areas. So, by the end of the nineteenth century the aphasiology data was pointing convincingly to the LH as the neurological locus for language. This led to *Localization Theory*—the view that specific functions had precise locations in the brain. A corollary to this theory was the notion of *Cerebral Dominance*—the view that the LH was the dominant one for generating the higher forms of cognition. Although the origin of this term is obscure, it grew no doubt out of the research connecting language to the LH and out of the cultural link in Western society between language and the higher mental functions. It took the subsequent research in neuroscience most of the first half of the twentieth century to dispel the notion that only the verbal part of the brain was the dominant one, and to establish the fact that the brain is structured in such a way as to provide for two modes of thinking, the verbal and the nonverbal. As the historians of neuroscience Springer and Deutsch (1993: 23) aptly put it, *Cerebral Dominance Theory* nicely captured the idea of "half a brain directing thought and behavior." This is why for most of the first half of the twentieth century the LH was designated a "strong" hemisphere, and the RH, in contrast, a "weak" or "minor" hemisphere.

But ever since its formulation, Cerebral Dominance Theory had dissenters. The nineteenth-century British neurologist John Hughlings Jackson (1874, 1878)—paradoxically one of the congeners of the dominance notion—was already casting doubts on the extreme view inherent in strict Cerebral Dominance Theory by pointing out that patients suffering from Broca's aphasia were nonetheless able to carry out basic communicative interactions, and by suggesting that reading might involve the RH.

In 1929, the American psychologist Karl Lashley (1890-1958) questioned the validity of localization method generally, claiming that while the origin of a particular function can perhaps be traced to a specific brain site, its overall modality (manifestation and characteristics) involved other sites. In the 1930s, the Russian psychologist Lev S. Vygotsky (1896-1934) argued, further, that language in a restricted sense—i.e. as phonemes, words, and grammatical categories—did indeed have a primary locus in the LH; but as a communicative-expressive modality it was more likely to arise from various synaptic connections that were distributed throughout the brain. Vygotsky suggested, moreover, that the whole brain, not just one hemisphere, was endowed at birth with a unique kind of "plasticity" that rendered it highly sensitive and adaptive to stimuli during childhood. Therefore, he put forward the intriguing proposal that localization processes were constantly being subjected to modifying influences from rearing, cultural, and other kinds of environmental factors. The brain, Vygotsky argued, was hardly a "hard-wired" mechanism; on the contrary, it was a highly adaptable and plastic organ.

Vygotsky's *Plasticity Hypothesis* became the point-of-departure for the work of another Russian psychologist, Alexander Luria (1902-1977), who in 1947 went even further in suggesting that there existed an interconnectivity in functional task distribution that spanned the entire brain. Adopting the linguist Roman Jakobson's (1942) idea that the *selection* of linguistic units and their *combination* were neurologically complementary processes, Luria showed that the latter was impaired by lesions in the anterior areas of the language centers, whereas the former were disrupted when damage occurred to the posterior areas of the same centers. Luria argued that although a single linguistic function (articulation, comprehension, etc.) could be safely located in a specific area of the LH, the overall phenomenon of language as an expressive and representational code resulted from the interaction of several cooperative cerebral structures that were connected by a network of synaptic processes. Subsequent aphasiology studies have confirmed Luria's basic idea: e.g. LH-damaged patients continue to use intonation patterns correctly (Danly and Shapiro 1982), suggesting a RH location for this function; RH-damaged patients, on the other hand, show little or no control of intonation (e.g. Heilman, Scholes, and Watson 1975, Ross and Mesulam 1979). Recent work on so-called *parallel distributed processes* (Rumelhart and McClelland 1986) has, in effect, been shedding some light on how Luria's idea of interconnectivity may in fact be the source of the higher mental functions.

Complementary Hemisphericity Theory

It was during the 1950s that the final blows against Cerebral Dominance Theory were delivered by the widely-publicized "split-brain" studies conducted by the

American psychologist Roger Sperry (1913-1994) and his associates. Split-brain patients—known more technically as *commisurotomy* patients—were epilepsy victims who had had their two hemispheres separated by surgical section of the corpus callosum in order to attenuate the seizures they tended to suffer. Each of their hemispheres could thus be "investigated," so to speak, in isolation by simply presenting stimuli to them in an asymmetrical fashion. So, any visual or audio stimulus presented to the left eye or left ear of a split-brain subject could be assessed in terms of its RH effects, and vice versa any visual or audio stimulus presented to the right eye or right ear could be assessed in terms of its LH effects. The commisurotomy studies were pivotal in providing a detailed breakdown of the main psychological functions according to hemisphere. And by extension, they suggested that in the "intact brain" both hemispheres, not just a dominant one, were needed in a neurologically-cooperative way to produce complex thinking abilities. The split-brain experiments established, in a phrase, that the two hemispheres complement each other in normal cognitive processes. The main L-Mode and R-Mode functions they established are well-known today:

Table 1. Modal Functions

L-Mode Functions	R-Mode Functions
major speech subsystems (pronunciation, grammar, etc.)	intonation and other prosodic subsystems
literal meaning	metaphorical, and emotional meaning
sequential relations	spatial relations
verbal memory	nonverbal memory
logical thinking (deduction, induction, etc.)	intuitive and spatial reasoning
abstracting and generalizing	concretizing and associating among things
analysis and linear thinking	synthesis and multiple thinking

This catalogue makes it obvious that in order to carry out a complex cognitive task (e.g. problem-solving in mathematics, discourse programming, reading, etc.) the integrated cooperation of both modes is required. Cognition, in other words, is *interhemispheric*, not just the product of dominant sites or centers in one or the other of the two hemispheres of the brain.

The use of clinical methods such as aphasiology data and of commisurotomy experiments as the primary *modus operandi* in establishing facts about brain functioning came under fire in the late 1960s. By the mid-1970s, neuroscientists started developing a host of non-clinical techniques to investigate the brains of normal subjects. Some are still in use today. They include dichotic listening (sending signals to the brain via headphones), electroencephalograph analysis (graphing brain waves with electrodes), and lateral eye movement (videotaping the movement of the eyes during the performance of some cognitive task). The findings generated by such techniques started casting further doubt on the idea that the LH alone was responsible for language. They showed, on the contrary, that the functions related to discourse programming—putting a message together to fit a situation, a topic, a need, etc.—were controlled by the RH or else were interhemispheric. By the early

1980s, the new experiments confirmed, for instance, that metaphor, intonation, verbal humor, and even some aspects of segmental phonology were controlled by the RH in tandem with corresponding centers in the LH.

Recent Trends

Such non-clinical techniques have been largely abandoned today for a simple reason—they have been made obsolete by new technologies such as *Positron emission tomography* (PET) scanning and *functional magnetic resonance imaging* (fMRI). These have enabled neuroscientists to observe the brain directly while people speak, listen, read, and think. These are particularly useful because they do not require any physical contact with the brain. They produce images similar to X rays that show which parts of the brain are active while a person carries out a particular mental or physical task. PET scanning shows the parts of the brain that are using the most glucose (a form of sugar), and fMRI shows the parts where high oxygen levels indicate increased activity.

The PET and fMRI studies are now confirming that language processing is extremely complex, rather than involving a series of subsystems (phonology, grammar, etc.) located in specific parts of the brain (Broca's area, Wernicke's area, and Penfield's area). The neuronal structures involved in language are spread widely throughout the brain, primarily by neurotransmitters, and it now appears certain that different types of language tasks activate different areas of the brain in many sequences and patterns. It has also become apparent from fMRI research that language is regulated, additionally, by the emotional areas of the brain. The limbic system—which, as we saw above, includes portions of the temporal lobes, parts of the hypothalamus and thalamus, and other structures—may have a larger role than previously thought in the processing of certain kinds of speech (Damasio 1994).

The *connectionist* views of Vygotsky and Luria are being largely corroborated by the new modes of neuroscientific investigation. This suggests that the brain is a highly *modular* organ, with each module (agglomeration of neuronal subsystems located in a specific region) organized around a particular task. The processing of visual information, for instance, is not confined to a single region of the RH, although specific areas in the RH are highly active in processing incoming visual forms. Rather, different neural modules are involved in helping the brain process visual inputs as to their contents. Consequently, visual stimuli that carry linguistic information would be converted by the brain into neuronal activities that are conducive to linguistic, not visual, processing. This is what happens in the case of American Sign Language (a gesture language for the hearing impaired). The brain first processes the meanings of visual signs, extracting the grammatical relations in them, in a connected or distributed fashion throughout the brain (Hickok, Bellugi, and Klima 2001). But visual stimuli that carry a different kind of information—such as the features of a drawing—are converted instead into neuronal activities that are involved in motor commands for reproducing the drawing. This finding would explain why tonemes (tones with phonemic value) are not processed by the RH, as it is the case for musical tones. Tone systems serve verbal functions, thus calling into action the LH. Musical tones instead serve emotional (aesthetic) functions, thus calling into action the RH.

The connectivity that characterizes neural networks has been examined not only experimentally with human subjects, but also theoretically with computer software. Computer models of the brain are called *Parallel Distributed Processing* (PDP) models. These are designed to show how, potentially, brain networks interconnect with each other in the processing of information. The PDP models appear to perform the same kinds of tasks and operations that language does (MacWhinney 2000). As Obler and Gjerlow (1999: 11) put it, in the strong form of PDP theory, "there are no language centers per se but rather 'network nodes' that are stimulated; eventually one of these is stimulated enough that it passes a certain threshold and that node is 'realized,' perhaps as a spoken word."

The Neurolinguistic Methods

Does neuroscientific research have any implications for classroom SLT? I believe that it does, as do many other teachers. In my view, knowledge about the brain provides a solid theoretical basis upon which the reformist paradigm can be rebuilt to meet contemporary conditions and expectations. Tackling the SLT Dilemma without such knowledge—especially since it is so readily available today—would be unnecessarily narrow-minded and retrograde. As mentioned in the previous chapter, this very perspective was adopted by a number of pioneering language educators after the demise of the ALM. Using neuroscientific reasoning, they designed methods that, they claimed, would activate the brain in a learning-productive fashion. The most widely-known NLMs (Neurolinguistic Methods) that resulted from this updated reformist view of things were *Suggestopedia, Total Physical Response*, and the *Natural Approach.*

The founders of the NLMs consistently reported eye-opening results involving all types of learners. This notwithstanding, they have never really caught on with teachers broadly. In my view, the fundamental reason for this lies in the fact that they require the teacher's total commitment to their methodology and overall educational philosophy. This pedagogical insularity (which at times has bordered on the fanatical) has made it impossible to adapt the NLMs to different learning situations. As were the DM or the ALM before them, the NLMs are simply too dogmatic in their overall "view of things." Nevertheless, some of their pedagogical ideas have become used widely. Moreover, their basic view that SLT should be designed as a "brain-compatible" enterprise is now an implicit one in SLT circles generally.

Suggestopedia

Suggestopedia is the brainchild of the Bulgarian physician and psychotherapist Dr. Georgi Lozanov, who first proposed it in the 1960s. It is based on the hypothesis that SLA involves primarily subliminal (unconscious) R-Mode processes. To activate such processes, Lozanov introduced the *séance* into the classroom—a phase during which students perform yoga meditation, sitting comfortably in reclining chairs and listening to background classical music (usually the slow movements of Baroque composers), while the new language material is introduced.

The class size is limited to no more than 12 students (composed ideally of 6 females and 6 males). Lessons are designed to last four hours, six days a week. Each one is divided into three phases:

> Review
>
> During this phase the previous day's material is reviewed through the use of conversations, skits, and games. Mechanical exercises are also used if needed.
>
> Séance
>
> With students sitting in specially constructed chairs arranged in a circle, the teacher conducts yoga breathing and meditation exercises as the new material is introduced and rehearsed through dialogues. The students follow along with a written version of the new material, as they listen to Baroque music.
>
> Follow-Up
>
> The new material is explained in traditional ways. However, situational practice based on real life is used as well to complement the presentation. Emphasis is placed on vocabulary and content, not on complicated grammatical matters. However, grammar is not ignored, and various L-Mode techniques are used (e.g. explanation and translation) to impart knowledge of structure so that the student can grasp the new material at an analytical-reflective level of mind.

Asking the students to assume "new identities" is also part of Suggestopedia's methodology. As the course progresses, the students are, in fact, expected to take on an imaginary life—as if they were someone reared and living in the target culture. The dialogues used in the course are then progressively scripted to contain references to the "biographies" of the assumed personas of the students. This is, clearly, an ingenious way of personalizing the learning process, so that the students do not focus consciously on linguistic forms, but rather on how they can be used to convey Selfhood.

The séance and the strange terminology used by Lozanov has laid Suggestopedia open to much criticism in the West. As Richards and Rodgers (1986: 142) observed a little while back, "the method has a somewhat mystic air about it, partially because it has few direct links with established learning or educational theory in the West, and partially because of its arcane terminology and neologisms, which one critic has unkindly called a 'package of pseudo-scientific gobbledygook'." The séance is perhaps the main reason why its introduction into North American classrooms was delayed until the late 1970s, after Sheila Ostrander and Lynn Schroeder, in their book *Psychic Discoveries Behind the Iron Curtain* (Bancroft 1978), argued that it produced incredibly effective learning outcomes in Eastern Europe. In my view, the aspect of the séance that is particularly interesting is the use of background music, for the reason that music has been shown to engage the R-Mode in learning tasks of all kinds (Hachinski and Hachinski 1994, Holden 1994). However, caution is to be exercised in assuming that music is effective for all types of students. Some students would perceive music as distracting, rather than helpful.

Lozanov has been criticized above all else for not justifying the neuroscientific evidence from which he purportedly derived the technique of the séance. For example, no evidence can be found, to the best of my knowledge, to support his claim that only 4% of the brain is actually utilized during traditional language teaching. He refers to the areas that make up the remaining 96% as "reserves" of the mind. Presumably, the séance is designed to tap into these reserves.

But perhaps the greatest problem with Suggestopedia is the credibility of Lozanov's extravagant claims. He maintains that his method will produce unheard-of results after just 24 days of instruction. To quote Lozanov (1978: 321-322) directly:

> If we take the 24 days' foreign language course with four lessons a day as the basic patterns, the following results can be expected: (1) The students assimilate, on average, more than 90 percent of the vocabulary which comprises 2000 lexical units per course. (2) More than 60 percent of the new vocabulary is used actively and fluently in everyday conversation and the rest of the vocabulary is known at the translation level. (3) The students speak within the framework of the whole essential grammar. (4) Any text can be read. (5) The students can write, although making some mistakes. (6) The students make some mistakes in speaking, but this does not hinder the communication. (7) Pronunciation is satisfactory. (8) The students are not afraid of talking to foreigners who speak the same language. (9) The students are eager to continue studying the same foreign language and, if possible, in the same way.

Lozanov's claims can only be received with a large dose of skepticism, even though supporters of Suggestopedia are quick to come to Lozanov's defense (Bancroft 1978, 1995, Schiffler 1992). Suggestopedia has even inspired "spin-off methods" such as the ACT *(Acquisition through Creative Teaching)* method (Dhority 1992). However, as Stevick (1980: 230) perceptively wrote during the height of the Suggestopedia craze just over two decades ago, it is rather obvious that the claims made by Lozanov and his acolytes need to be investigated more thoroughly in order for their method to become more mainstream in SLT. The main questionable claims are:

- that a student learns much faster when his/her unconscious mind is activated;
- that subliminal processes *in all individuals* can be activated through meditation techniques and exposure to Baroque music;
- that learning is held back by failure to make use of the reserves of the brain.

The one thing that clearly makes sense, without much question, is Suggestopedia's insistence on establishing a congenial, relaxed learning environment. The research documenting the benefits of creating such an environment is rather straightforward and unequivocal (e.g. Schwartz, Davidson, and Maer 1975, Ostrove, Simpson, and Gardner 1990). A relationship of trust and respect between the teacher and the student is probably the best way to activate (rather than impede) the crucial emotional areas of the brain. The question vis-à-vis the séance, therefore, is not its unorthodox nature, but rather whether or not it actually activates these regions of the brain (as Lozanov claims). My suspicion is that it does and, hence, would explain why the method is apparently as successful as it is purported to be.

Whether or not Suggestopedia is as effective as Lozanov and other dedicated followers claim, is really a moot point—after all, other methods, approaches, and pedagogical movements have hardly produced any better results. However, although it does seem to suit certain types of learners, it is probably not effective with all learners in all situations. As was the case with the congeners of the DM and the ALM, Lozanov simply assumes that his pedagogical proposals are applicable to *all students, anywhere*, and at *any time*. This simply is not the case, as the history of SLT has shown time and time again.

Total Physical Response

Total Physical Response (TPR) was proposed by James Asher in 1964, a professor of psychology at San Jose State University. As Richards and Rodgers (1986: 34) stated in their 1986 survey of methods, TPR has always attracted a larger following of teachers than Suggestopedia because it draws on several familiar Western traditions, "including developmental psychology, learning theory, and humanistic pedagogy, as well as on language teaching procedures proposed by Harold and Dorothy Palmer."

TPR is based on four central R-Mode principles:

- Receptive skills emerge before productive skills.
- A close relationship between instructor and learner will minimize the inhibitions and fears that impede language acquisition.
- The new SL input should be imparted with verbal cues that get students involved in physical activities.
- New material should be introduced only when the students are capable of understanding what it allows them to do.
- If the new input is not learned rapidly, then students are obviously not ready for it. Consequently, it should be withdrawn and presented again at some future time.

When a sufficient amount of R-Mode learning has taken place, Asher affirms, the L-Mode will be triggered *on its own* to produce grammatical abstractions. For this reason, grammar training is not employed in TPR. Asher bases this claim on brain physiology. As we saw above, the somatosensory cortex receives messages from the sense organs as well as signals from all parts of the body and the environment. If stimulated with R-Mode techniques involving physical activity, Asher believes that this region of the brain will trigger association and memory regions in tandem. In effect, the brain will analyze and store linguistic information *autonomically* when properly "activated" through R-Mode techniques.

The physical activities in TPR are linked to imperative verb forms and general command protocols in the SL. This type of input is similar to what children are exposed to in NLA: e.g. "Give mummy your hand;" "Sit down;" "Eat your dinner;" etc. Clearly, Asher espouses the same SLA = NLA theoretical view that the congeners of the DM did. But, even though learning a language through actions does indeed facilitate the acquisition process, there are other techniques that can accomplish the same kinds of learning goals that these are designed to realize. Moreover, my own practical experiences reveal that some (perhaps most) adult learners often refuse to become involved physically in the classroom, as if they were children. And this may be the reason why TPR has never quite worked its way into the pedagogical mainstream. Like Suggestopedia, it is not applicable to *all learners* in *all learning situations*.

The Natural Approach

In 1977, the late Tracy D. Terrell, a professor of Spanish linguistics and a brilliant instructor of SLs (as I was able to witness myself on a number of occasions), proposed the *Natural Approach* (NA). By the early 1980s Terrell started collaborating with Stephen Krashen, an applied linguist at the University of Southern California. Together, they refined NA into a method which, for a time, became one of the most discussed teaching proposals in SLT generally, given its intuitive appeal to teachers and learners alike. Like Suggestopedia and TPR, the NA also ascribed great salience to the R-Mode during all stages of SLA, but especially during the initial ones. And like TPR, it deemed explicit grammar training to be practically useless, since it posited that knowledge of structure would emerge autonomically through the brain's inbuilt "monitoring" system. However, before his untimely death in the early 1990s, Terrell (1991) modified this dubious view considerably. Unfortunately, since his death, NA has virtually disappeared from the SLT "radar screen."

The NA was based directly on Krashen's *acquisition-learning* dichotomy (chapter 1). From an analysis of interlanguage data, Krashen (1985: 1) arrived at the conclusion that the former typically unfolds through a "natural sequence:" i.e. students acquire certain structures before others. And this, he claims (1985: 1), "does not appear to be determined solely by formal simplicity;" nor is it dependent on "the order in which rules are taught in language classes." More than anything else, it is triggered spontaneously by the learning environment itself. As Krashen put it, students typically bring an "affective filter" to the learning process—a mental block that prevents them from fully acquiring the comprehensible input to which they are exposed. When it is "up" (i.e. when they are unmotivated, lacking in self confidence, or anxious) they may understand what they hear and read, but they will not be able to *acquire* it. When the filter is "down," however, they are not hampered emotionally by the possibility of failure. When acquisition is set in motion, then *learning* the rules of grammar, Krashen (1985: 1-2) claims, will take place as the need arises:

> Acquired competence comes from our subconscious knowledge. Learning, or conscious knowledge, serves only as an editor, or Monitor. We appeal to learning to make corrections, to change the output of the acquired system before we speak or write (or sometimes we speak or write, as in self-correction). I have hypothesized

> that two conditions need to be met in order to use the Monitor: the performer must be consciously concerned about correctness; and he or she must know the rule.

The primary strategy in getting acquisition to unfold *naturally* is to ensure not only that the input to which learners are exposed is understandable, but also that it contains "a bit" of information that is beyond the student's developing competence (Krashen 1985: 2):

> The Input hypothesis claims that humans acquire language in only one way —by understanding messages, or by receiving "comprehensible input." We progress along the natural order by understanding input that contains structures at our next "stage"—structures that are a bit beyond our current level of competence. We move from i, our current level, to $i + 1$, the next level along the natural order, by understanding input containing $i + 1$. We are able to understand language containing unacquired grammar with the help of context, which includes extra-linguistic information, our knowledge of the world, and previously acquired linguistic competence.

Whether or not the NA has the capacity to produce the significant learning outcomes that Krashen and Terrell assumed would ensue from its utilization continues to be a matter of debate. Like TPR, it was based on the belief that SLA occurred in the same neural pathways of the brain as NLA. But the evidence used in support of the SLA = NLA hypothesis has always been anecdotal or based solely on pedagogically-persuasive argumentation, not on any strict neurological evidence. No faultfinding is intended here because there really is no way to confirm or disconfirm this hypothesis, short of using PET-scanning equipment on students throughout a course of study. Judiciously, Krashen and Terrell have always claimed that their views were based on anecdotal evidence and on pedagogical tradition, rather than on strict neurological research. And this, in my view, is all that can ever be done in the search for insights from the neuroscientific domain

Neurolinguistic Questions

Suggestopedia, TPR, and the NA were the first serious attempts in the history of SLT to base classroom pedagogy on the view that the brain's acquisition mode—the R-Mode—is the crucial one in SLA. In so doing, however, they downplayed the role of the L-Mode perhaps too drastically. They continue to generate much interest and enthusiasm in teacher and learner alike during the initial stages—the stages during which the R-Mode probably dominates the intake of novel information. But their overemphasis on this mode throughout the course of SLA also probably explains why, by the early 1990s, interest in them declined considerably. With the advent of the Proficiency Movement (chapter 1) a few years later, they came to be viewed as too "fixated" on their specific idiosyncratic view of SLA—the same fanatical fixation that brought about the downfall of all previous methods.

The NLMs were instrumental, nevertheless, in focusing or refocusing attention on four critical neurolinguistic issues. These are (1) the SLA = NLA hypothesis, (2) the CPH issue, (3) the role of the RH in SLA, and (4) the usefulness of UG Theory for SLT.

The SLA = NLA Hypothesis

As discussed in the previous chapter, the hypothesis that spawned the Reform Movement in SLT was that SLA = NLA. But, to the best of my knowledge, no neurolinguistic evidence has ever cropped up to support this hypothesis. Lamendella (1977, 1979) claims that the available evidence suggests, on the contrary, that NLA takes advantage of innate neural systems that are available only up to puberty. The Canadian linguist Michel Paradis (1987: 131) similarly suggests that the native and second language (learned after puberty) are "subserved by different neural circuits at the micro-anatomical level."

But despite such interpretations of the relevant data, it is likely that the SLA = NLA hypothesis is partially correct. Adolescent and adult SL learners do indeed manifest many of the same acquisition patterns that children do during NLA. It is a self-evident fact that learning a second language, after puberty, will enlist many of the same neurological resources involved in childhood language acquisition. But it is also true that SLA in adulthood will entail other processes, as the transfer theorists pointed out during the ALM era. Indeed, there is now evidence in the neurosciences that there may be neurologically-differentiated linguistic and conceptual systems that are involved in the transfer process. That will be the topic of the fourth chapter.

The CPH Issue

Lenneberg's CPH hypothesis, as discussed, claims essentially that the brain loses its capacity to transfer the language functions in aphasics from the LH to the nonverbal RH after puberty, which it was able to do, to varying degrees, during childhood. The CPH appeared to receive support early on from a widely-reported case of a child, named Genie, whose abusive father had isolated and physically restrained day and night in a small bedroom with little light and virtually no stimulation from the age of 20 months (Curtiss 1977). When found at almost the age of 14, and thus after the critical period, as Lenneberg's CPH predicted Genie could not speak, nor was she ever able to learn how to speak like someone who had had the benefit of a normal upbringing. However, many doubts have been cast on using Genie's case as supporting the CPH. As Obler and Gjerlow (1999: 72) put it: "Genie's case was not an ideal one for testing what happens with late language acquisition because there is some question as to whether she was mentally retarded from birth and thus her father was responding so cruelly to her abnormal development. The extreme deprivation that she suffered also may have had biological influences on her brain, so it is unlikely that we see in her simply an example of 'normal' delayed language acquisition."

Lenneberg's time frame was hotly contested by SL teachers almost from the outset. Krashen (1973, 1975), for instance, concluded, *on the basis of the same data* used by Lenneberg, that the critical period occurred much earlier (by around 4-5 years of age), thus implying that factors other than neurological ones are involved in the apparent decrease in the capacity of adolescents and adults to acquire native-like competence in another language. Perhaps the most exhaustive critique of the CPH has come from the pen of Thomas Scovel (1988) who, in reviewing the extensive body of research evidence assessing the CPH, reached the conclusion that there are no clear-cut findings to suggest biological constraints on SLA. Lenneberg, as Scovel points out, simply assumed that language acquisition was easier for children. Moreover, since the CPH really has implications for the acquisition of pronunciation, rather than for other kinds of SL skills, at the very least it should be recast to take this into account. As Seliger (1978) and Walsh and Diller (1981) have suggested, perhaps there are many critical periods corresponding to the various levels, or subsystems, of language.

A few studies have actually suggested that older children and adolescents do better than younger children at certain aspects of the SL in a natural environment. Cognitive maturity in older learners would appear to allow them to deal with the more abstract aspects of language and "context-reduced types of tasks" (Harley 1986: 15). Krashen pointed out that older learners' knowledge of the world would make input more meaningful and comprehensible to them than to children. Older learners' interpersonal skills also allow them to participate more actively and efficiently in conversations; they thus succeed in acquiring sufficient input from conversations.

There are many variables besides biological factors and cognitive maturity that could affect a learner's success in the acquisition of the SL. These include affective, personality, cognitive, and many others. In effect, studies have yet to prove any direct relationship between age difference and the learner's success in the acquisition of the SL. We certainly need more evidence in this field in order to interpret the implications of the CPH more precisely.

The Role of the RH in SLA

Since the 1970s, it has become clear that the LH is not the only locus for language. The research has shown rather conspicuously that the RH plays a complementary role in speech. The relevant findings can be summarized in chart form as follows:

Table 2. Modal Speech Functions

Main L-Mode Functions Involved in Speech	Main R-Mode Functions Involved in Speech
phonology	prosody (rhythm, intonation, etc.)
morphology and syntax	iconicity (onomatopoeia, rhyme, etc.)
anaphora and deixis (substitution processes)	implication (statement vs. question, suggestion vs command, etc.)
literal meaning	figurative meaning
sentence structure	message meaning

This pattern of hemispheric complementarity suggests that the L-Mode is responsible for the relations inherent among the structures that make up the various sentences of a speech act, whereas the R-Mode is responsible for the expressive and signifying properties inherent in the act itself. Speech is, in effect, an interhemispheric phenomenon. Generally, the RH controls metaphorical and connotative meaning (Winner and Gardner 1977, Brownell 1988, Danesi 1989, Rapcsak, Beeson, and Rubens 1991) and many areas of discourse programming (e.g. Behrens 1989, Hough 1990, Kaplan, Brownell, Jacobs, and Gardner 1990, Rayman and Zaidel 1991). The LH, instead, controls grammar, morphology, literal meanings, and segmental phonology—although Segalowitz and Cohen (1989) found evidence to suggest that even some aspects of phonology may involve both hemispheres, not just the LH.

The research on the RH led some language educators in the early 1980s to propose a *stage model* of SLA (e.g. Obler 1980, Galloway and Krashen 1980)—a proposal which assigned a dominant role to the R-Mode during novel learning tasks. Supporting this model was a key study published in 1981 by Goldberg and Costa. The two neuroscientists suggested that the RH is a crucial point-of-departure for novel tasks because of its anatomical structure. Its greater connectivity with other centers in the complex neuronal pathways of the brain makes it a better "distributor" of new information. The LH, on the other hand, has a more sequentially-organized neuronal-synaptic structure and, thus, finds it more difficult to assimilate information for which no previously-formed synaptic circuits exist. Pedagogically, this suggests that for any new input to be comprehensible, it must allow the synthetic functions of the RH to do their work first. The NLMs, as we saw above, were implanted on this fundamental principle.

At this point a caveat is in order. The exaggerated claims made by those who subscribe to "right-brain" educational models are products of a social trend. The "discovery" of the RH by neuroscience during the split-brain era was interpreted by many socialist philosophers and media pundits as vindicating the view that Western education was biased in favor of the LH, i.e. in favor of analytical, deductive, and rational thought at the expense of creative, imaginative, and intuitive thinking. This led, shortly thereafter, to what Gardner (1982: 266-267) aptly characterizes as "the temptation to tamper with the work of scientists," and consequently to a tendency to put forward sensational claims about "right-brain learning" by a coterie of "academic hucksters," as Gardner calls them. Educational constructs derived from neuroscience, although highly plausible, are nonetheless artificial ones. Unless they lead to calculable results they are worthless in and of themselves.

UG Theory

The neuroscientific focus in SLT has opened up a meaningful debate on the implications of Universal Grammar (UG) Theory, if any. The UG is, supposedly, an innate tendency that equips humans by the age of two to utilize a set of "rule principles" to develop the specific "rules" (known as "parameters") of the language to which they are exposed. This would purportedly explain the universality and rapidity of NLA. Indeed, UG theorists claim, the only requirement for learning any language is adequate exposure to samples of it from birth to about two, and full language will emerge through the operation of the UG's set of principles. As Chomsky (1986) cleverly put it, language is as natural to the human being as flight is to a bird. The way a bird flies is irrelevant; what is important is that all birds are "destined" to fly—for that is their nature. The implication is that all languages are built from the same basic neural blueprint and that differences among them are explainable as choices of rule types from a fairly small inventory.

As mentioned in the previous chapter, the problem with UG Theory is that it ignores the role of imitation and of the nonverbal faculties in NLA. The cognitive scientist Philip Lieberman (2000) even argues that, as an overarching theory of language, it is useless because it posits syntactic rules as the set of principles that make up the UG. What about other aspects of language structure? And how did syntax come about in the first place? Lieberman suggests that language is an extension of sensory processes. The linguist Ronald Langacker (e.g. 1987, 1990, 1999) agrees, arguing that the extension comes about to displace sensory processes. Take, for instance, nouns. With our eyes we perceive things as having or not having *boundaries*. This perceptual feature is precisely what nouns are designed to encode by extension. Thus, for example, the noun *leaf* encodes a bounded referent, whereas the noun *water* encodes an unbounded referent. This perceptual dichotomy has consequences in the domain of grammar—*leaves* can be counted, *water* cannot; *leaf* has a plural form *(leaves)*, *water* does not (unless the referential domain is metaphorical); *leaf* can be preceded by an indefinite article *(a leaf)*, *water* cannot; and so on. Similar perceptual codifications can be found in other representational systems—in painting, for instance, *water* is represented either with no boundaries or else as bounded by other figures (land masses, the horizon, etc.); *leaves,* on the other hand, can be depicted as separate figures with circumscribable boundaries. This suggests that grammatical rules are hardly present in the brain at birth but, rather, that they are extensions of sensory processes.

Grammar is, Langacker asserts, a strategy for organizing our direct perception of things in the world as they stand in relation to one another. Consider the relation between an active and passive sentence: e.g. *Alexander ate the apple* vs. *The apple was eaten by Alexander.* When the subject (*Alexander*) is in the *foreground* and the object (*apple*) in the *background*, the active sentence is used. It encodes a *view* of the subject as a "perpetrator" of some action (*eating*). A change from passive to active entails a shift in *viewing*. The passive sentence brings the *apple* to the foreground, relegating the eater *Alexander* to the background. The action of *eating* is now spotlighted on the object, the "receiver" of the action. In effect, passive sentences encode a different mental angle from which the same action can be seen.

Langacker's "perception-extending grammar" theory—which is called rather appropriately *Cognitive Linguistics* today—constitutes a good account of how sentence composition reflects experience of the world. This is probably why language and the ability to draw emerge in tandem in the child. The child learns early on that language allows him/her to a model and reflect upon the world in the same way that a drawing or a melody does. In the same way that a painting is much more than an assemblage of lines, shapes, colors, and melodies a combination of notes and harmonies, a sentence in language is much more than an assemblage of words and phrases built from some rule system in the brain. We employ grammatical elements at our disposal to model the world in ways that parallel how musicians use melodic elements and painters visual elements to model it.

In SLA circles, UG Theory has been the target of much research of late. It has been used by some to explain why SLA is so arduous after puberty. Presumably, the UG in the brain has "done its job" by then. Others argue that the UG will continue to operate after puberty, under certain conditions. Suffice it to say for our purposes that the work on UG Theory in SLA has produced very little of value in the domain of pedagogy. As we saw in the previous chapter, the only method that has incorporated the basic blueprint of Chomskyan grammatical theory in the past was the Cognitive-Code Method. However, the interesting feature of that method was hardly the way in which it treated grammar, but how it interrelated linguistic structure with meaning. Paradoxically, the nature of that very interrelation is something that has always been a thorn in the sides of generativists, and it continues to be debated heatedly within UG theoretical circles to this day.

CHAPTER 3
MAKING SECOND LANGUAGE TEACHING "BRAIN-COMPATIBLE"

The most important part of teaching = to teach what it is to know.

Simone Weil (1909-1943)

Introduction

As we saw in the previous chapter, neuroscience has now established that the brain's two hemispheres differ not so much as to the type of stimuli they are designed anatomically to process, as to the manner in which they process information. This is why it is improper, if not misleading, to use terms such as "right brain learning" or "left brain ideas." There are no such things. Terms such as "L-Mode" and "R-Mode," on the other hand (Edwards 1979), are preferable because they refer only to types of processes associated with one or the other hemisphere. The PET-scanning research has shown that while each hemisphere is specialized to handle a certain specific type of function, it does so in tandem with complementary or parallel processing patterns taking place in the other hemisphere (and in other parts of the brain). So, the term "R-Mode" is used in this book to refer to functions that have a primary locus in the RH, but which activate other areas of the brain in an interconnected fashion. Similarly, the term "L-Mode" is used in reference to functions whose neural substrate is in the LH, but which stimulate other areas of the brain in an interdependent fashion. But as adaptable and neuroscientifically-consistent as such terminology is, its incorporation into SLT begs the following question: Is there any pedagogical advantage in using such terminology?

Danesi and Mollica (1988) attempted to answer this very question, examining the viability of utilizing terms such as "R-Mode" and "L-Mode" to help guide instructional practices. They trained teachers of two high schools in the Toronto area how to prepare their instructional practices in line with Bimodality Theory—i.e. by viewing certain techniques as R-Mode, L-Mode, or intermodal, and then organizing their classes according to a set of four basic "modal principles" (which will be discussed in this chapter). As it turned out, at the end of the academic year, the two experimental high school classes fared significantly better on all tests of proficiency than did two control classes taught according to a standard communicative syllabus. But the significant finding of the study was not so much the difference in proficiency levels obtained, as the fact that teachers could be easily trained to organize their pedagogical routines by adopting a specific "brain-compatible" view of SLT—Bimodality Theory. Soon after the study was published, the researchers realized, however, that the results could be explained in non-neuroscientific ways.

One could say, for instance, that the bimodally-trained subjects achieved higher proficiency levels for the simple reason that they were taught by techniques that were varied and sufficiently well-designed *in themselves*. This would preclude any need to explain the positive results in terms of neuroscientific concepts. The study thus raised a rather fundamental question for this whole line of inquiry: To what extent is it meaningful to label a technique, *X*, as R-Mode, and another one, *Y*, as L-Mode? It is difficult to see how to gather empirical data to answer such a question. But perhaps it is a moot one, after all. The value of such terminology lies not so much in predicting what parts of the brain may or may not be activated, as it does in furnishing insights for organizing SLT *in a general way*; i.e. it is useful insofar as it leads to effective ways of structuring classroom input, designing syllabuses, and doing all the things that are required for carrying out SLT in a classroom environment.

In effect, the Danesi and Mollica study showed that neuroscientific constructs could have pedagogical consequences. Follow-up work (e.g. Lombardo 1988, Nuessel and Cicogna 1992, Pallotta 1993, Arnò 1993, Schenone 1994, Curro 1995, Smor Forster 1995) has provided both empirical and anecdotal support of this general finding. The objective of this chapter is, therefore, to discuss the kinds of pedagogical principles that can be envisioned by considering the relevant brain research with this objective in mind. In my view, there are four such principles that are worth considering. These can be called as follows: (1) the *modal flow principle*; (2) the *modal focusing principle*; (3) the *contextualization principle*; and (4) the *conceptualization principle.*

Incidentally, before dealing with these principles, it is interesting to note that the notion of bimodality provides a convenient "diagnosis" of why so many methods and approaches in SLT have tended to come and go. Simply put, it suggests that any instructional system that privileges one or the other of the two modes is bound to fail sooner or later. Such a system can be called *unimodal*. For the most part, the techniques that were molded into inductivist and deductivist methods (the GTM, the DM, the ALM, etc.) focused on developing L-Mode control of the SL. It was assumed, on the whole, that the ability to synthesize and apply L-Mode functions to carry out communicative tasks would emerge spontaneously in the learner. In all fairness, it should be acknowledged that some of the techniques used within the framework of the inductivist methods—e.g. the use of situational practice, the incorporation of visual stimuli, the contextualization of practice routines, etc.—did have an R-Mode focus. And this might, in fact, explain why they have survived to this day as effective techniques *on their own*. But it still remains true that the overall instructional design of the inductivist methods was L-Mode. On the other side of the unimodal continuum, Communicative, Humanistic, and Neurolinguistic methods and approaches were designed with an opposite unimodal bias. They typically overemphasized the R-Mode to the detriment of the L-Mode. This is why they always generated much interest and enthusiasm at first, but seldom produced high levels of proficiency by the end of a course of study.

Needless to say, no one method or approach has ever been designed intentionally to be unimodal. It is more accurate to think of SLT practices generally as placeable on a continuum with two extreme endpoints: an L-Mode, or extreme analytical point, and an R-Mode, or extreme experiential point. The midpoint of this continuum is, in effect, the "breakpoint" at which an SLT practice takes on more and more of the modal characteristics of that half of the continuum as it approaches an endpoint. Thus, for instance, the Grammar-Translation Method, in its extreme form, would be located at the L-Mode endpoint; Silent Way teaching, on the other hand, would be placed at the R-Mode endpoint; communicative approaches that integrate formal skills into their instructional plan would be located near the breakpoint but slightly to its right; and so on.

Two Modal Principles

Before discussing any principles derived from a neuroscientific view of pedagogy, it is necessary to clarify the meaning of the word *theory* in *Bimodality Theory*. In no way does it imply a "theory" in the usual scientific sense—e.g. as in the *theory of light*, the *theory of the atom*, etc. It constitutes, simply, a speculative plan as to how instruction in the SL classroom might be carried out, based on a set of underlying neuroscientific principles that have been verified to some degree by actual classroom experience and research. Bimodality Theory constitutes a specific *view* of SLT that is derived from a consideration of the relevant hemisphericity research—the original Greek meaning of *theory* was "view." It *sees* the brain's experiential and analytical modes of acquiring knowledge as systematic contributors to SLA in its totality—as a tool for constructing narratives, for evoking humor, etc. As Gardner (1981: 74) has aptly put it: "Only when the brain's two hemispheres are working together can we appreciate the moral of a story, the meaning of a metaphor, words describing emotion, and the punch lines of jokes."

The Modal Flow Principle

As teachers know all too well, students will absorb new material much more readily and meaningfully if they are given opportunities to *do* something with it. When this typical observation is mapped against the relevant neuroscientific work on hemisphericity, a "perfect match" results. In a phrase, it would seem that for the brain to take in unfamiliar information it requires the experiential (probing) R-Mode functions to operate freely. However, both the anecdotal experiences of teachers and the neuroscientific findings also indicate that this exploratory effort on the part of students would be virtually wasted if not followed up by the teacher's "analytical" intervention, so to speak. All this suggests a general *principle* of language learning:

> *The Modal Flow Principle*
>
> New notions and structures are learned more efficiently when the learner's brain is allowed to process it in terms of an R-Mode (experiential) to L-Mode (analytical) "flow."

The main pedagogical implications of this principle are rather straightforward. During the initial learning stages, students need to assimilate input through observation, induction, simulation, oral tasks, and various other kinds of R-Mode experiential activities. But after this "orientation stage," students must be exposed to formal grammatical explanations, practice drills, and other kinds of L-Mode techniques. The *modal flow principle* thus claims that: (1) experiential forms of tutoring belong to the initial learning stages; (2) teaching should become progressively more formal and analytical after these stages; and (3) the creative utilization of the new input belongs to the final stages. Stage (1) can be called simply an R-Mode stage, stage (2) an L-Mode stage, and stage (3) an intermodal stage:

R-Mode stage →	**L-Mode stage →**	**Intermodal stage**
Experiential learning of new input through orientation tasks	*Formalization and practice of new input*	*Utilization of new input in creative ways*

Figure 5. Modal Flow

An analogy to music teaching can perhaps be made here to illustrate the practical implications of this principle, not to mention its validity as a construct for explaining all types of learning situations. Learning how to play a new piece on the piano, say, entails the ability to mold the component mechanical skills needed to play the notes, phrases, etc. of the piece successfully into the global skill of "playing the music." So, in order to give the learner's L-Mode a better opportunity to organize the component skills into automatic psychomotor routines, the teacher normally starts out by playing the piece for the student, making appropriate aesthetic comments here and there, relating these to the techniques needed to successfully execute the new piece. In this way, the student's R-Mode has an opportunity to decipher the new musical input in a global aesthetic way. The component mechanical skills can then be understood separately and practiced apart from their expressive modalities. Needless to say, an advanced piano student who is already in firm control of the required L-Mode skills through previous training will not have to spend as much time on this orientation phase as would a beginner. When the student has mastered the L-Mode aspects of the piece, then he/she will be in a position to integrate them with the R-Mode ones as he/she performs the piece. A consummate performance of the piece is, from a neurological perspective, an *intermodal* feat, requiring the integrated contribution of both the R-Mode and the L-Mode to the performative task at hand.

The modal flow principle makes one fundamental demand on the teacher—it requires the teacher to identify a specific learning task as being novel or not. Generally speaking, something is novel when it involves structures or concepts that are either different or absent from the NL linguistic and/or conceptual systems. More will be said about this below and in the next chapter. Suffice it to say at this point that any task or input can be considered to be "novel" if the students demonstrate an inability to understand it or use it functionally right away. If that is so, instructional techniques that focus on discrete categories (explaining words in isolation, elucidating rules of grammar, etc.) will be of little value, since the students have no preexisting L-Mode schemas for accommodating the new information directly. In order to make something accessible to the L-Mode, pedagogical experience dictates that the learner should be allowed to explore the new structures and concepts through R-Mode techniques (dialogues, questioning strategies, simulation activities, etc.). Once the initial R-Mode orientation stage has been allowed to "run its course," the teacher must "shift modes" and put the student in a frame of mind that allows him/her to reflect on the new structural patterns *in themselves*. This implies the use of L-Mode techniques such as grammatical explanations, mechanical exercises, etc. Only after it can be ascertained that the students have become familiar with the structural and conceptual features of the new material should they be allowed to use these creatively and meaningfully in communication tasks. This "intermodal stage" is a point of arrival that is reached at different times by different learners. There is no way to predict when a certain student will reach it; but when he/she does it is obvious to teacher and learner alike. As in Asher's TPR approach, that is the point at which the next novel task or input can be introduced efficiently to that learner, without interrupting the learning flow that has been established.

Obviously, this means that time-based courses of study will have to be adapted to the modal flow principle. Generally speaking, however, time differences in learning need not be perceived as disruptive of general classroom procedure. Students who reach the intermodal stages more slowly than others, should be given much more individual attention, with R-Mode or L-Mode techniques as the case may warrant. The others can be assigned various individualistic intermodal tasks (writing, reading, etc.) that will allow them to utilize their time functionally, as the slower learners "catch up."

The modal flow principle can be seen to be a different version of the oldest principle in SLT—the *inductivist principle*. But unlike its use in strictly inductivist methods (e.g. the DM, the ALM, etc.), it does not require that induction training be employed for *all* learning tasks; only those that involve new information or novel orientation tasks. Thus, if a learning task contains knowledge or input that the learner already recognizes, the modal flow can be efficiently avoided. So, this principle is really a common-sensical pedagogical notion that good teachers, and the more effective SLT methods, have always utilized in their *modus operandi*. It is virtually a "law of learning" which claims that teaching should ensure a constant flow from experiential to formal learning tasks and from practical to theoretical content. Indirect evidence in support of the modal flow principle exists throughout the SLA and SLT literatures. Jeffries (1985), for example, has shown that the use of grammatical rules to start a new unit of learning (an L-Mode practice) poses a serious obstacle to classroom acquisition. And the recent literature on communicative methodologies scattered throughout the SLT journals suggests that the overemphasis on R-Mode techniques in the last three decades has greatly undervalued the role of grammatical training and practice drills.

There are many R-Mode techniques that can be used to facilitate and promote initial learning efforts. Dialogues are a case in point. As the great methodologists of SLT history knew, these allow students to become familiar with the new input in an experiential way. Even though the dialogues prepared by the methodologists were often artificial, i.e. strictly-controlled for grammar and vocabulary, the dialogue format nevertheless provided a stimulus for the student to explore new meanings and new modes of expression *in his or her own way*. For this reason, dialogues are extremely useful during the initial R-Mode stage in the learning flow. The teacher should allow for much improvisation on the part of students and encourage them to participate in the performance of a dialogue. Instructional techniques that focus on discrete categories in the dialogue (the meaning of words in isolation, the morphological characteristics of verbs, etc.) will have little impact on learning outcomes, since the students generally have no preexisting L-Mode schemas for accommodating such information directly. Nevertheless, the teacher should relay what new words mean (using the NL of the student if necessary), so that the flow is not disrupted in any significant way. Glosses can also be used to expedite matters.

Consider, as a case-in-point, the following mini-dialogue, which has been written to simulate the ways in which beverages are ordered at an espresso bar in Italy:

Sarah:	*Un caffè, per favore.*	("A coffee, please.")
Barista:	*Come lo desidera?*	("How would you like it?")
Sarah:	*Lungo.*	("Mild"/"Long.")
Barista:	*EccoLe!*	("Here you are!")
Sarah:	*Grazie.*	("Thank you.")
Barista:	*Prego.*	("You're welcome.")

To allow the R-Mode to grasp the information *in its own way*, students can be asked to provide variations to the dialogue by extemporizing and adding their own versions to its basic format, no matter how many structural errors they might commit in the process. The actual time it takes for this cognizing stage to run its course will depend on the learners themselves (i.e. on the kind of linguistic know-how they bring to the classroom, on their previous familiarity with Italian coffee, etc.).

Now, in order for the new structures and concepts in the dialogue to reach long-term memory, this R-Mode stage must be followed up by techniques that allow the student to reflect and analyze the new content—e.g. by comprehension exercises (*Che caffè desidera Sarah?* "What type of coffee does Sarah want?"), explanations of the new vocabulary and grammar items, etc. This secondary stage in the flow cannot be circumvented. L-Mode knowledge simply will not emerge on its own, as Asher or Krashen (among others) apparently believed (chapter 2). Obviously, some types of learners will need fewer formal explanations and exercise reinforcement practice than others. Moreover, the type of L-Mode instruction to be used will vary according to both learner cognitive style and type of input—some tasks are best taught through inductive procedures, others through deductive ones. The way to determine what L-Mode technique is appropriate is simply to try one out. Clearly, if a deductive technique doesn't seem to work, then an inductive one (or a different deductive one) must be considered. Similarly, the degree of utilization of the student's NL during L-Mode instruction will depend on the level of competence reached by the learners—the more the students are familiar with the SL the more the new material can be explained without translation. Commentaries on any pattern or feature related to, or derived from, the new content should be elaborated when required. In the above dialogue, therefore, information on politeness vocabulary (*grazie, prego*, etc.) and on the social differences between *tu* and *Lei* (familiar and polite pronouns of address) should be highlighted.

Finally, after the formal practice of the new material in the dialogue has taken place, and it is obvious that students can control it conceptually and structurally, then they can be allowed to use it creatively—e.g. ordering coffee in different preparations, showing politeness to other students in the class, etc. This intermodal stage thus puts the ball back into the students' court, so to speak. It is only during this stage that role-playing, group work, and other communicative techniques will produce meaningful results—*not before*, as has been assumed by communicative methodologists. The intermodal stage involves *recognition*, i.e. the ability to use previously-acquired knowledge to decipher and participate in unscripted conversation. It is also during intermodal stages that supporting texts—a piece of realia, an excerpt from the work of some important writer, etc.—can be used profitably to extend learning in an $i + 1$ fashion, as Krashen characterizes this crucial aspect of SLA (chapter 2).

The general operational procedures that the modal flow principle entails can be summarized as follows:

During an R-Mode Stage

- Classroom activities should be student-centered.
- Students should be allowed to explore the new material through experiential activities (dialogues, simulations, etc.).
- Each student should be encouraged to participate in the activities, unless, of course, a shy student refuses to do so. In the latter case, the learner should be allowed to participate whenever he/she feels ready to do so (or else to grasp the new material individualistically).

During an L-Mode Stage

- The focus is on the teacher.
- The teacher should explain the structural and conceptual features of the new material clearly using deductive or inductive techniques as warranted by the situation.
- Any notion that the students appear to have difficulty grasping should be reinforced with appropriate comparisons to the NL and with suitable exercise material.
- Oral and written exercises, pattern drills, etc. should be used to reinforce what has been learned.

During an Intermodal Stage

- The learner should be allowed to employ the new material to carry out real-life verbal tasks, but only after he/she shows the ability and willingness to do so.

- Teaching new things or discussing matters of form and structure during this stage should be avoided.
- Students should be allowed to find solutions to problems of communication on their own. As in Di Pietro's Scenario Approach (1987), the learners should be encouraged to generate their own strategies for orchestrating role-playing scenarios. The teacher should act as adviser and guide to individuals or groups as needed.
- Role-playing and work in pairs or groups is advisable for most students, although some may not wish to participate. The latter can be assigned other kinds of creative tasks (e.g. writing).

As mentioned above, the modal flow principle is derived, first and foremost, from classroom experience. But it is consistent with the neuroscientific research on hemisphericity which, as we saw in the previous chapter, strongly suggests that the R-Mode is a crucial point-of-departure for activating the appropriate language acquisition areas of the brain. This is because the RH is an effective distributor of new information. It is an *efferent* hemisphere, designed anatomically to transmit impulses from its various neuronal networks to others throughout the brain. The LH, on the other hand, with its more sequentially-organized neuronal-synaptic structure, is an *afferent* hemisphere, designed anatomically to receive impulses rather than transmit them.

The Modal Focusing Principle

At various points in a course of study, individual students may manifest some persistent difficulty in utilizing a feature of grammar, vocabulary, etc. At other points, they may show difficulty in using a certain speech act in conversations or in saying something in a conceptually-appropriate fashion. At such points, it is obvious that they will need to *focus* on form, meaning, or function, as the case may be. This aspect of SLA can be called *modal focusing*:

> *The Modal Focusing Principle*
>
> It is necessary from time to time in a course of study for the student to focus on some modal feature or pattern that is causing him/her difficulty.

When a learner needs help in overcoming some grammatical error pattern that has become an obstacle to learning, then "L-Mode focusing" techniques must be used to allow that student an opportunity to relearn the grammatical feature in question. "R-mode focusing" techniques, on the other hand, may be needed when a student shows the inability to apply a certain concept or structure in discourse or text-construction. In essence, this principle claims that in any course of study there will be points when the student may need to stop and focus on certain aspects of the material introduced for which he/she manifests a need to reinforce or relearn. It derives, clearly, from the common observation of teachers that students typically need to get more practice in doing such things as conjugating verbs correctly (L-Mode focusing), using speech formulas in appropriate ways (R-Mode focusing), etc.

A comparison with music teaching can again be made in order to emphasize the crucial role that modal focusing plays in all kinds of learning situations. The best way to teach a music student how to play a new piece of music, as mentioned above, is to do so in line with the modal flow principle. Now, as the student starts practicing the new piece of music, he/she might experience some specific technical difficulty during the execution of a certain passage. The reason for such difficulty might be that the practice routines he/she executed previously were insufficient, that he/she never really mastered the scale on which that passage is constructed, that the way in which he/she integrated the passage to the other parts of the piece was faulty, etc. Whatever the case may be, the student will obviously have to stop playing the piece in its entirety and focus on the passage in question, working on it until he/she overcomes the difficulty he/she has in executing it proficiently. Without such L-Mode focusing, the ultimate performance of the piece would be impaired by technical inconsistencies or flaws. On the other hand, the student might need to focus on some aspect of expression or phrasing that is getting in the way of a successful aesthetic execution of the piece (R-Mode focusing). In such a case, the student will need to "re-experience" the aesthetic qualities of that passage by listening to his/her teacher play it again.

From a neurological standpoint, different hemispheric learning styles—a predisposition for one or the other learning mode due to personality or background factors (Geschwind and Galaburda 1987)—will always have to be taken into account in the design of focusing techniques, and tailored accordingly. It is obvious that students with a dominant L-Mode learning style will need to understand what they are doing more so than will those with a dominant R-Mode style. As teachers know all too well, some students want to understand everything they are learning; others instead seem to be content with grasping things casually. More than likely, this is because the former are L-Mode-dominant, and the latter R-Mode-dominant.

A "hemispheric profile" of learners can easily be drawn up as a framework for indicating the kinds of modal focusing techniques that would be appropriate for specific types of learner. Simply put, those with an L-Mode-dominant style will need to be given more explanations and drills during focusing stages. Those with an R-Mode-dominant style will generally not need as many of these. Needless to say, only the day-to-day contact with learners will allow teachers to figure out what probable hemispheric style an individual student may possess. The following chart contains the main characteristics that are associated with each modal style. These have been compiled from extensive work on both brain patients and normal subjects. It should be pointed out, however, that such "dichotomies" are a bit artificial, in that very few humans (if any) really fit the profile. It is more accurate to say that the traits given below are dominant in some individuals rather than in others, but that every individual has both kinds of traits 9to greater or lesser degrees). Moreover, life experiences—including training in a classroom—can essentially modify the individual's brain to assume more of his/her nondominant traits, thus becoming more "bimodal" in overall cognitive style. Bimodality is, thus, an objective that can be imparted to anyone, no matter what his/her dominant hemispheric style:

Table 3. Modal Learning Style

Individual with an L-Mode-Dominant Learning Style...	Individual with an R-Mode-Dominant Learning Style...
is less willing to talk spontaneously, and rarely takes the initiative in conversations	is more willing and able to engage in conversation, and generally takes the initiative in discussions
Shows a good control of basic vocabulary, but a poorer overall ability to use vocabulary creatively	Shows a richer and more varied vocabulary
Uses grammatical forms accurately, after having learned them thoroughly	is more inclined to use grammatical forms spontaneously, even before he/she controls them
is generally inclined to be careful about his/her speech appropriateness	is inclined to ignore error in speech
Perceives speech sounds individually (is good at spelling and pronunciation)	is aware mainly of entire words
is less capable of extracting the meanings inherent in the novel verbal material	Has a greater comprehension ability of novel verbal input
His/her intonation patterns tend to be dull	His/her intonation patterns tend to be more lively
is more capable of memorizing abstract grammatical concepts.	is more inclined to memorize meanings rather than individual grammatical concepts.
is not good at body language.	is excellent at body language.

The Contextualization Principle

Memorizing or pronouncing words in isolation, or rehearsing speech formulas without reference to some situation that typically entails them, is rarely conducive to learning—no matter what one's dominant hemispheric learning style may be. The reason is, simply, that language derives its meaning potential from the *contexts* in which it occurs or to which it refers in usage. Without sufficient context, it is unlikely that the brain can assimilate new input in any mnemonically-functional way. Essentially, during an R-Mode stage, the brain requires the kind of conceptual information that will allow it to decipher the cultural references which the new material can evoke. During an L-Mode stage, on the other hand, the brain requires practical or conceptual information to complement its analytical efforts:

> *The Contextualization Principle*
>
> During an R-Mode stage, the new material must contain references to cultural concepts in order for the brain to detect the appropriate meaning potential of the new structures; during an L-Mode stage, the practice and re-

hearsal of the new structures is greatly enhanced if practical or conceptual information is provided.

Much work has been done on contextualization techniques since the mid-1980s (e.g. Omaggio 1986, Shrum and Glisan 1994). Essentially, these are of two types: (1) *cultural contextualization* techniques, which are designed to provide culturally-appropriate information during an R-Mode stage; and (2) *practical contextualization* techniques, which are designed to provide similar information during an L-Mode stage.

Cultural Contextualization

Cultural contextualization techniques provide information that allows students to relate the novel linguistic input to cultural concepts, symbolism, rituals, etc. The word *context*, incidentally, derives from Latin *contextus* "connection," which, in turn, comes from *cum* "with, together" and *textus* "fabric." It literally means "together with a *text*," alluding to the fact that any meaningful verbal text constructed in a language is tied to some aspect of the cultural conceptual fabric from which it is cut. The dialogue above, for instance, included several items of information that rendered it culturally meaningful:

- a reference to a type of Italian coffee (*espresso)*;
- a reference to a type of coffee preparation *(lungo)*;
- an exemplification of politeness strategies *(per favore, Come lo desidera? EccoLe, Grazie, Prego).*

In effect, the contextualization principle asserts that novel input must contain references to cultural information whenever possible, otherwise it will produce few learning effects. Sometimes, the information may have to allude to variation in the SL. In northern Italy, for instance, there is a tendency to use the present perfect to describe virtually all past actions—e.g. *Sono andato al cinema la settimana scorsa* "I went to the movies last week." In many parts of southern Italy, the tendency is, instead, to use the past absolute—*Andai al cinema la settimana scorsa.* Referring to a "watermelon" as *cocomero, anguria,* or *melone* also falls along regional lines: *cocomero* is used primarily in central and south-central parts of Italy, *anguria* in northern Italy, and *melone* in many parts of southern Italy. Such variation is an intrinsic part of Italian discourse expectancy.

Practical Contextualization

Practical contextualization refers to the use of meaningful information or reference to realistic situations in the design of exercises and activities used during an L-

Mode stage. For example, conjugation exercises involving the imperative tense should give the student a sense of how the verb forms can be used practically. Here is a simple example of contextualization involving this tense in Italian:

> Your father wants to lose weight, so an Italian doctor gives him some advice. Provide the doctor's commands as suggested.
>
> Model *mangiare meno* ("to eat less")
> *Mangi meno!* ("Eat less!")
>
> 1. *cominciare una nuova dieta* ("to start a new diet")
> 2. *uscire una volta al giorno* ("to go out once a day")
> 3. *fare ginnastica* ("to work out")
> 4. *camminare invece di guidare* ("to walk instead of to drive")

There are the many suggestions in the SLT literature for creating contextualized practice exercises and activities. There is no need to give a detailed breakdown of these here. The main ones are as follows:

> *Culture-Focused Contexts*
>
> These allow students to carry out the practice of forms, conjugations, etc. in culturally-focused ways:
>
> Order the following beverages (coffee, tea, etc.)
> Make a deposit at a bank of $500 dollars
>
> *Situational Contexts*
>
> These allow students to relate the forms, conjugations, etc. to situations:
>
> Ask the person next to you what her favorite beverages are and why.
> Ask how much something costs.
>
> *Identification Contexts*
>
> These require students to identify specific facts using the new forms, conjugations, etc.
>
> What is the name of a certain person?
> Where does he/she come from?
>
> *Function-Related Contexts*
>
> These involve getting students to relate the forms, conjugations, etc. to speech functions:
>
> Form questions asking the following things...
>
> where Sarah goes to school

what Alexander is doing tonight

Personalized Contexts

These involve getting the learners to use the forms, conjugations, etc. to express personal points of view in a controlled manner:

Say whether you do or do not like Italian coffee.
Indicate how to say hello.

Information-Giving Contexts

These involve getting students to use the forms, conjugations, etc. to convey culturally-appropriate information:

Say what kind of dwelling an Italian would live in.
Give a typical Italian address.

Information-Getting Contexts

These involve getting students to use the forms, conjugations, etc. to get culturally-appropriate information:

Ask a partner what radio or TV program is currently popular in Italy (if he/she knows).
Ask your friend if he/she knows what the time is in Italy at this moment.

Cultural Identification Contexts

These require students to recognize certain facts about the SL culture as they use the forms, conjugations, etc.:

Give the Italian for each of the following—five well-known movie directors, five great artists, etc.
Name five Italian car models.

Cloze Tasks

These require students to supply words that were systematically deleted from an SL text (an article from a newspaper or magazine, a cartoon strip, etc.). Such texts require the student to glean the indicated form from the contextual information provided by the text.

Description Tasks

These require students to describe certain things or people using the forms, conjugations, etc. to refer to cultural things:

Describe what an Italian might wear to go to university, to go out at night on a date, etc.
Name five colors that describe what you are wearing.

Open-Ended Completion Tasks

These require students to finish certain statements logically:

The euro is diminishing because...

Problem-Solving Tasks

These require students to use the forms, conjugations, etc. to solve problems of communication:

How would you say hello in Italian?

The Conceptualization Principle

A common observation of teachers is that students often produce SL messages that are "semantically anomalous" when they attempt to speak or write spontaneously, without some form of guidance. The source of such anomaly is, typically, the unconscious tendency of students to put together SL messages on the basis of NL concepts. This topic will be discussed in detail in the next chapter. Suffice it to say here that this common tendency of learners suggests a fourth general principle:

The Conceptualization Principle

When students create an SL message on their own, they tend to "think" the message out in terms of their NL conceptual system. The result is a message that is structurally Italian, French, Spanish, etc. (the SL), but conceptually English (the NL). The teacher must thus ensure that the two systems—the linguistic and the conceptual—are interrelated during all aspects and stages of instruction and practice.

Concepts serve classificatory functions. Some are universal. Distinguishing, for instance, between *living* and *nonliving* things, between *people* and *animals*, between *males* and *females*, and so on constitute categories that serve basic practical functions for people cross-culturally. But many others are culture-specific. Distinguishing between kinds of snow will have a high conceptual priority for those living in cold climates. That is why there are many words for snow in Inuit and indigenous Scandinavian languages, but very few (if any) in languages spoken by people living in warm climate zones.

The psychologist Elinor Rosch (1973a) has suggested that there are three levels of such "distinction-making:"

- *superordinate*, which involves distinction-making at a highly general classificatory level—e.g. *feline, equine, human, animal*, etc.;
- *basic*, which involves distinction-making at a practical typological level —e.g. *cat, tiger, lion*, etc. are types of *felines*;

- *subordinate*, which involves distinction-making at a detail-providing level—e.g. *Siamese, tabby,* etc. are species of *cats*.

Concepts do not exist in a vacuum. They derive their functions in relation to other concepts and systems of reference. Consider, for example, what happens when we look up the definition of a word such as *cat* in a dictionary (Danesi 2000). Typically, the latter defines a *cat* as "a carnivorous mammal (*Felis catus*) domesticated since early times as a catcher of rats and mice and as a pet and existing in several distinctive breeds and varieties." The problem with this definition is that it uses a superordinate concept *mammal* to define a basic one, *cat*. What is a *mammal*? The dictionary defines *mammal* as "any of various warm-blooded vertebrate animals of the class Mammalia." What is an *animal*? The dictionary goes on to define an *animal* as "a living organism other than a plant or a bacterium." What is an *organism*? An *organism*, the dictionary stipulates, is "an individual animal or plant having diverse organs and parts that function together as a whole to maintain *life* and its activities." But, then, what is *life*? *Life*, it specifies, is "the property that distinguishes living organisms." At that point the dictionary has gone into a conceptual loop—i.e. it has employed an already-used concept, *organism*, to define *life*.

Looping is caused by the fact that definitions employ words, which of course encode other concepts, to define a specific concept. One way around this is to use imagery—e.g. a drawing or a photograph of a cat—as do so-called *visual dictionaries*. But this technique creates problems of a different nature (e.g. Which image or photo is the appropriate one culturally?). As it turns out, the dictionary approach is the only possible one. All human systems of knowledge have a looping associative structure. This suggests that the meaning of something can only be inferred by relating it to the meaning of something else to which it is associated. There simply is no such thing as an "absolute concept." So, the meaning of *cat* is something that is extrapolated from the chain of associated concepts that it evokes. In addition to the concepts of *mammal, animal, organism*, and *life*, used by the dictionary, one can add subordinate ones such as *whiskers* and *tail* to the "associative chain."

Concrete Concepts

There are two main types of concepts. In both philosophy and psychology, they are called *concrete* and *abstract.* A *concrete* concept is one that refers to something that can be pointed out in some physical way. *Cat* is an example of a concrete concept. As another example, consider the meaning of the word *blue* in English. It refers to a hue on the color spectrum with a wavelength of approximately 450 to 490 nanometers. The specific image that comes to mind will be different from individual to individual. But all images will fall within the above wavelength. The concept of "blueness" is forged by observing the hues found in natural phenomena such as the sky and the sea. Concrete concepts allow speakers of a language to talk and think about perceivable things in specific ways. They are not universal, necessarily. The color terms used by one language group will vary from those used by another. There are many historical reasons for this. It is not necessary here to engage in a discussion about the universality or relativity of concrete concepts. Suffice it to say, that what seems like a "natural category" to one culture (e.g. "blueness"), may not seem so natural to another, which may find it sufficient to distinguish between "dark" and "light" hues for practical purposes (as is the case of the Bassa language spoken in Liberia).

Abstract Concepts

Concrete concepts are rather limited when it comes to serving the need of describing emotions, morals, ideas, etc. For such purposes, *abstract* concepts are employed. These refer to things that cannot be demonstrated in some physical way—e.g. *sadness, secrecy, personality, justice*, etc. How do you point out *sadness* or *secrecy*? Rather than "pointing out" such things, languages use their resources to "represent them" in some imaginative way. Consider, for instance, the use of *cat* and *blue* in the following sentences:

1. Jack's a real cool *cat.*
2. Today my sister has the *blues.*
3. My brother let the *cat* out of the bag.
4. That bit of news hit me right out of the *blue.*

These sentences show that abstractions are conveyed typically by the process of *metaphorical association*. The use of *cat* in (1) to mean "attractive," "engaging," etc. comes out of the discourse associated with jazz music; and the use of *blues* in (2) to mean "sad," "gloomy," etc. comes out of the tradition of blues music talk. The use of *cat* in (3) to convey "secrecy" and the use of *blue* in (4) to convey "unexpectedness" also have historical traditions behind them. In our culture, cats are perceived as secretive beings and are often portrayed as such in language and other representational systems. Sentence (3) is, in effect, a specific instantiation of the conceptual metaphor *animals reflect human life and activities*, which underlies common expressions such as:

5. It's a *dog's* life.
6. Your life is a *cat's* cradle.
7. I heard it from the *horse's* mouth.

Sentence (4) is also an instantiation of a conceptual metaphor—namely, *Nature is a portent of destiny.* Literary critics classify this metaphor as a stylistic technique under the rubric of *pathetic fallacy*. This underlies such common expressions as:

8. I heard it from an *angry wind.*
9. *Cruel clouds* are gathering over her life.

Like concrete concepts, therefore, the meanings of abstract concepts also emerge through *association*. But it is not one based on *association-by-sense*, as it is in the formation of the former. Rather, it is based on *association-by-inference.*

This is an R-Mode function, as the vast literature on RH processing in semantics shows (e.g. Ardila 1984, Brownell 1988, Chiarello 1988b, Joanette, Goulet, and Hannequin 1990, Kaplan, Brownell, Jacobs, and Gardner 1990, Hunter and Liederman 1991, Beeman 1993, Bottini et al. 1994). To grasp what this means, consider the word *tail*, which the dictionary defines as "the flexible appendage found at the rear end of an animal's body." This is the concrete meaning of *tail*, providing basic information about what a *tail* is—an extremity—and where it is found on an animal—on its rear end. Now, these details are what guide the extension of *tail* to encompass meanings such as following:

10. The *tail* of that shirt is not bleached.
11. Do you want heads or *tails* for this coin toss?
12. The *tail* section of that airplane is making a funny noise.

Such associations are hardly random or disconnected to the original concrete concept. Shirts, coins, and airplanes are inferred in English-speaking cultures as having appendages and rear ends. In conceptual terms, a *shirt*, a *coin*, and an *airplane* are things that belong to separate categories of their own. However, through associative inference they are interlinked to the *tail* concept.

Implications

The conceptualization principle has several pedagogical implications. Above all else, it suggests that conceptual knowledge cannot be separated from knowledge of either *langue* or *parole*. The *langue-parole* dichotomy was introduced into linguistics by Ferdinand de Saussure (1916), who used the analogy of a chess game to illustrate what it entails. To engage in a game of chess both players must first know the *langue* of chess—the rules of movement and the overall strategy of how to play. *Langue* imposes constraints on, and provides a guide to, the choices each player can make in the act of playing the game. The actual choices characterize *parole*—the ability to apply the abstract knowledge of chess *(langue)* to a specific game-playing situation.

The structuralist methods in SLT emphasized knowledge of *langue*, believing that the ability to apply them to communication (*parole*) would emerge on its own. Rarely did those methods entertain how to relate *langue* to the concepts it encompassed systematically. On the other side of the methodological coin, the communicative approaches focused on the development of *parole*, believing that knowledge of *langue* would be induced by the learners themselves. However, they too rarely entertained how to relate *parole* to the concepts that speech acts manifested systematically. So, in effect, both types of approaches ignored the conceptualization principle in their *modus operandi*.

To grasp the main difference between the structuralist and communicative approaches, consider the treatment that the partitive structure in Italian would receive hypothetically by each one. The partitive is composed of the preposition *di* and the various forms of the definite article which are inflected according to the gender, number, and initial sound of the following noun (or adjective):

dei libri	("some books")
delle matite	("some pencils")
degli studenti	("some students")
della carne	("some meat")

In a structural syllabus this structure would be introduced only *after* the prepositions, articles, and rules of contraction had been learned and reinforced:

di + i = *dei*
di + le = *delle*
di + gli = *degli*
di + la = *della*
etc.

In a communicative syllabus, on the other hand, the partitive would be introduced whenever it was required in the given sequence of functions to carry out some communicative task. Its structural features would be discussed at that point, whether or not students had been exposed to prepositions, articles, and/or rules of contraction:

Function: ordering food and beverages

Io prendo della carne ("I'll take some meat").
Vorrei del caffè ("I would like some coffee").
etc.

Function: buying things

Maria vuole comprare delle matite ("Mary wants to buy some pencils").
Voglio dei libri ("I want some books").
etc.

Students taught by either approach, however, experienced considerable difficulty in knowing when and how to use the partitive (Danesi and Di Pietro 1991). The most likely reason for this was that they had not been taught to perceive a relationship between the concept of *partiality* and the forms that allowed speaker to utilize this concept in actual situations. In a phrase, they had not been taught to "think" of the partitive as part of the conceptual domain associated with nouns. They had been taught either to control its morphology (in structuralist approaches) or else to use it formulaically in controlled situations (in communicative approaches). The conceptualization principle implies, on the other hand, that such "conceptual knowledge" should be made available systematically through instruction. The appropriate "conceptual rule" that relates the partitive and the concepts it encompasses can be elaborated as follows. In Italian only singular forms of the partitive are used with mass nouns because one can only think of things such as "meat," "wine" etc. as "parts" of some "whole." On the other hand, only plural forms are used with count nouns because the latter evoke images of "countable things" such as "books" and "pencils:"

With mass nouns

Voglio della carne ("I want some meat").
Prendo del vino ("I'll take some wine").
etc.

With count nouns

Ho comprato dei libri ("I bought some books")
Hanno comprato delle matite ("They bought some pencils")
etc.

The central task facing students is, clearly, that of grasping such conceptual distinctions and how they are encoded by the SL morphology. Learning a new word, a new expression, or a new point of grammar implies, *unavoidably*, learning a new way of conceptualizing something.

Take, as another example, the task of learning SL words that resemble NL words in form, but have different meanings. These are called *deceptive cognates*, but are known more colloquially as *false friends*. In Italian, the word *sensibile* is not equivalent in meaning to the English cognate *sensible* ("rational"); in Italian it means "sensitive." Again, the primary task facing SL learners is a *conceptual* one. In this case, the domain is semantic, rather than morphological.

In developing "conceptual rules" for classroom purposes, it is important to keep in mind that conceptualization can unfold in one of three ways: (1) it can be *isomorphic*, whereby the forms of the NL and the SL reflect virtually the same conceptual structures; (2) *overlapping*, by which the forms have overlapping domains of meaning and use; and (3) *differentiated*, whereby they encompass completely different conceptual domains. A case of isomorphism can be seen, for example, between the word *car* in English and *automobile* in Italian—leaving out differences that occur at the level of cultural interpretation, since an Italian *automobile* evokes different perceptions than does an American *car*. Isomorphism is rare. Even among phylogenetically-related languages (e.g. English and German), it is exceptional to find concepts covering the same stretches of meanings exactly. More than likely, there will be some overlap between the conceptual domains, as we saw above in the case of English and Italian partitive structures. Differentiated concepts are, of course, the more problematic ones—e.g. explaining the uses of the Italian subjunctive to an English-speaking student, given that the subjunctive has largely disappeared from the English language (except in some specific usages).

The most difficult task facing learners, however, is not grasping conceptual differences in themselves, but rather how these are encoded in grammatically and lexically appropriate ways. This is an L-Mode task and implies teaching the forms and rules of the language code in a way that allows students to see how they relate to the concepts they encode. Various pedagogical suggestions for doing this will be discussed in the next two chapters.

The conceptualization principle implies that some errors (perhaps many) can be classified, not as *linguistic* or *communicative*, but *conceptual*. Consider the following erroneous sentences that were committed by students in my classes of Italian at the University of Toronto:

1. **Io aspetto per Maria ogni giorno* (intended meaning: "I wait for Mary every day").
2. **Ciao professore, ti vedo domani* ("Good-bye professor, I'll see you tomorrow").
3. **Io sono molto sensibile quando spendo soldi* (intended meaning: "I'm very sensible when it comes to spending money").
4. **Il gusto del caffè espresso è più che buono; è delizioso* (intended meaning: "The taste of espresso coffee is more than good; it is delicious").
5. **Io sono caduta in amore un anno fa* (intended meaning: "I fell in love a year ago").

Example (1) contains an error caused by a difference in syntax. In English, the verb *to wait* is intransitive and thus takes an indirect object preceded by the preposition *for*. In Italian, on the other hand, *aspettare* is a transitive verb and, therefore, takes a direct object without a preposition. Thus, (1) is a *linguistic error* caused by negative transfer at the level of sentence structure. Sentence (2) contains, needless to say, a purely *communicative error*—the use of the informal register of address with a professor. The last three examples contain *conceptual errors*. The students who uttered (3) and (4) assumed that the meanings of *sensibile* and *delizioso* were isomorphic to English *sensible* and *delicious*—but they are not. Example (5) contains an error in metaphorization. The student assumed that the conceptual metaphor *love is a trap* manifests itself in exactly the same way in the vocabulary choices of Italian—but again it does not.

Conceptual errors abound in student discourse (Russo 1997, Danesi 2000). They are the most difficult kind to detect. Consider the following two Italian sentences:

Sapevo che arrivava ieri ("I knew he was arriving yesterday").
Ho saputo che è arrivato ieri ("I found out he arrived yesterday").

Comparing these sentences with their English counterparts shows that Italian encodes "knowing" with one verb, *sapere*, capturing the difference between "knowing" and "finding out" in the past as a tense dichotomy. The former meaning is rendered by the imperfect form of the verb (*sapevo*) and the latter by the present perfect form (*ho saputo*). English, on the other hand, encodes the two concepts with separate words, thus assigning a separate category status to each one. This difference is the source of conceptual errors such as the following ones committed by two students of English at the University of Lugano whose NL is Italian (Danesi 2000):

*I *have known* that she called yesterday.

*I *was knowing* that they were studying.

Concepts are not encoded only in terms of grammatical and lexical processes, but by all the subsystems of a language. In English tonal distinction is not critical in conceptualization. It is, however, in North Mandarin Chinese which encodes numerous concepts by differences in the rise and fall of tone. The single syllable /ma/, for example, can have various meanings according to whether the tone is level (—), rising (↑), dipping (↕) or falling (↓):

/ma —/	"mother"
/ma ↑/	"hemp"
/ma ↕/	"horse"
/ma ↓/	"scold"

In English, tone is used for a different reason—to signal differences in discourse function. Statements, for instance, end with a falling intonation pattern; whereas some types of questions—e.g. those that can be answered with a *yes* or a *no*—end with a rising intonation pattern:

Do you speak English? (↑)

Do you know Ms. Jones? (↑)

Revamping Contrastive Analysis

The foregoing discussion makes it obvious that an expanded use of contrastive analysis (CA) will be necessary in a comprehensive approach to SLT. CA was developed, as mentioned in chapter 1, by audiolingual methodologists in order to determine what target and native language structures were similar and different in order to organize the teaching syllabus according to a simple learning principle—areas of similarity require less instructional emphasis and can be assumed to be acquired spontaneously, while areas showing differences require attention proportional to the degree of difference.

In its original form, therefore, CA came to be accepted both as a theory of SLA and as an organizing principle around which to plan for language teaching. As Stern (1983: 46) aptly put it: "Contrastive Analysis was not intended to offer a new method of teaching; but it was a form of language description which was particularly applicable to curriculum development, the preparation and evaluation of teaching materials, to the diagnosis of learning problems, and to testing." CA methodologists viewed the NL as a "filter" that was used by the learner for deciphering target language input.

It was the structural linguist Charles Fries (1927, 1945) who first developed CA during the 1940s, claiming that the unconscious transfer of NL grammatical and lexical patterns to the learning of the SL produces characteristic errors in those areas where such patterns are divergent or nonexistent. Fries' techniques were expanded by his student Robert Lado (1957) and, a little later, by a widely-acclaimed book series edited by Charles A. Ferguson, published by the University of Chicago Press (Kufner 1962, Stockwell and Bowen 1965a, 1965b, Agard and Di Pietro 1965a, 1965b).

In the late 1960s, however, CA was severely critiqued as the theoretical *Zeitgeist* in which it was developed—structuralism—gave way to cognitivism. As Wardhaugh (1970) pointed out, in its *strong* version, the Contrastive Analysis Hypothesis (CAH) was unrealistic because it claimed to be an *a priori* predictive theory of learning difficulties. Evidence emerged suggesting the exact opposite (Wode 1976), namely that dissimilarity between the NL and the SL might facilitate SLA, while similarity was more likely to lead to hamper it. Wardhaugh suggested that a more acceptable, *weaker* version could be employed to explain difficulties on an *a posteriori* basis. It was the late Robert J. Di Pietro (1971) who resuscitated interest in the weaker version of CA in the 1970s. By the 1980s, CA was expanded to encompass discourse analysis (e.g. James 1980, Fisiak 1981). The 1970s and early 1980s also saw the emergence of *Error Analysis* (chapter 1). Errors in student interlanguages were explained by error analysts as due to gaps in linguistic and/or communicative competence (e.g. Richards 1971, 1975, Corder 1971, Nemser 1971, Selinker 1972). The regular appearance of such forms as **he goed* and **she comed* in the interlanguages of foreign students of English could not be explained by transfer theory. These were explainable, rather, as resulting from overgeneralization—i.e. from the tendency to apply a rule learned previously to all the items of a linguistic category. Some SLA researchers (e.g. Dulay, Burt, and Krashen 1982) went so far as to claim that all errors, including those thought previously to have been caused by transfer, were the result of over- and undergeneralization. Others saw transfer and generalization as different sources of interlanguage errors. As Sridhar (1981: 232) put it: "Interlanguage takes all systems into account, explicitly incorporating the contrastive analysis of the learner's Interlanguage with both his native and the target language, the difference being that, in interlanguage, the contrastive analysis is an initial filtering device, making way for the testing of hypotheses about the other determinants of the learner's language" (see also Robinett and Schachter 1983, Faerch, Haastrup, and Phillipson 1984).

Despite critiques of its theoretical foundations, CA has shown itself to be a highly useful technique to this day. But it needs to be revamped because, in my view, its true value lies in allowing teachers to identify conceptual errors which, as Russo (1997) has documented, are the most prevalent ones in interlanguages. The reason for this is the fact that the student's native conceptual system is "the only system in previous experience upon which the learner can draw," as Brown (1987: 177) has so aptly put it.

In a revamped CA, therefore, the emphasis would be on showing how grammar, vocabulary, prosody, etc. reflect underlying conceptual structures. As a concrete example, consider how color terms can be introduced in a classroom situation. The connotative concepts encompassed by these can be included as part of a unit dealing with emotions. A CA of Italian and English, in this conceptual domain, would show differences such as the following:

Table 4. Color Concepts

Color terms	NL equivalents	Figurative uses	NL equivalents
arancione	orange	--	--
azzurro	blue	*il Principe azzurro*	Prince Charming
bianco	white	*notte bianca*	sleepless night
colore	color	*tutti i colori*	lot of trouble
giallo	yellow	*giallo dalla rabbia*	extremely angry
grigio	gray	*vita grigia*	dull life
marrone	brown	*fare un marrone*	make a big mistake
nero	black	*umore nero*	dark mood
rosa	pink	*acqua di rosa*	superficiality
rosso	red	*diventare rosso/a*	become embarrassed
verde	green	*al verde*	(financially) broke
viola	violet, purple	--	--

A simple exercise such as the following one can then be designed to bring out conceptual differences:

Fill-in the blanks with appropriate color terms:

Role A: *Anche tu sei di umore _____ (nero)*?
("Are you in a dour mood too"?)

Role B: *Eh, sì! Sono quasi sempre al _____ (verde) e faccio una vita _____ (grigia). E tu cosa fai?*
("Oh yes! I'm always broke and I live a dull life. What's with you?")

Role A: *Niente. Ultimamente, mia sorella ne sta facendo di tutti i ______ (colori)! Ieri mi ha fatto passare una notte _____(bianca)! È stata quasi tutta la notte al telefono con il suo Principe _____ (azzurro). Mi fa diventare ______ (giallo) dalla rabbia!*
("Nothing. Lately my sister has been causing a lot of trouble. Yesterday she made me go through a sleepless night! She was on the phone with her Prince Charming through the night. She makes me red with anger"!)

Students can then be asked to change the conceptual effect of certain colors in the above dialogue. For instance, the last sentence in the dialogue can be changed in several ways to make it more forceful:

> *Mi fa diventare collerico!* (literally: "She makes me become choleric")
>
> *Mi fa diventare pallido dalla rabbia!* (literally: "She makes me become pale with anger")

Once students have discovered the conceptual similarities and differences, they can be involved in reinforcing them through traditional pattern practice, translation, role-playing, and other such activities. In effect, imparting *conceptual competence* is not much different than imparting communicative or linguistic competence. It will just take more time and effort to do so.

The acquisition of new SL categories enlists higher-level conceptual systems, which can be stored as automatic subroutines at lower levels of encoding. In actual language performance, lower-level subroutines can be enlisted without calling upon higher-level ones. So, in conformity to current neurolinguistic theory, the conceptualization principle claims that the SL learner is faced with the task of identifying the encoding system best suited for the delivery of a conceptual task. In my view, the modal flow principle should be able to activate the appropriate regions and subregions of the brain involved in conceptualization, while modal focusing can entrench the relation between encoding and conceptualization, as needed. The problem lies, therefore, in identifying what is truly "novel" in the flow and what is not, in linguistic, communicative, and conceptual terms.

CHAPTER 4
FINE TUNING THE BRAIN FOR LANGUAGE ACQUISITION

If an educational act is to be efficacious, it will be only that one which tends to help toward the complete unfolding of life.

Maria Montessori (1870-1952)

Introduction

The research on the role played by the RH in language (Winner and Gardner 1977, Brownell 1988, Danesi 1989, Bottini et al. 1994), coupled with the general research on discourse in psychology and linguistics, has made it obvious that *metaphor* is a fundamental cognitive force in the etiology of human conceptual systems. As we saw in the previous chapter, it constitutes a central strategy in the delivery of abstract concepts. This aspect of conceptualization was investigated seriously by psychologists and linguists starting in the late 1970s. Their work has since led to the establishment of two significant new trends: (1) *Conceptual Metaphor Theory* (Lakoff and Johnson 1980, 1999, Lakoff 1987, Johnson 1987), and (2) a branch of linguistics that now comes under the rubric of *Cognitive Linguistics* (Langacker 1987, 1990, 1999, Allwood and Gärdenfors 1998, Dirven and Verspoor 1998).

The scientific work on metaphor has definite implications for SLT (e.g. Danesi 1993c, 1994b, MacLennan 1994, Russo 1997, Cameron and Low 1999), and will thus constitute the topic of discussion of this chapter. Perhaps the most important implication is that it suggests concrete ways of "fine tuning" the student's brain for acquiring *conceptual competence*, by making it sensitive to the conceptual structures that are required for the delivery of culture-appropriate abstract meanings in discourse.

Conceptual Competence

The research in Cognitive Linguistics suggests rather strongly that to be "conceptually fluent" in discourse is to know, in large part, how a language encodes abstract concepts on the basis of metaphorical reasoning. This kind of knowledge, like linguistic and communicative (pragmatic) knowledge, is by and large unconscious in native speakers. If a speaker of English were to talk about *time*, he/she would unconsciously employ conceptual domains that typically reveal metaphorical reasoning. For example, a statement such as "I have *spent* too much time on that project" reveals that he/she enlisted a metaphorical concept that has the general abstract form: *time is money*. Of course, the same speaker could have enlisted other metaphorical concepts—e.g. "That project is *wasting* my time;" "That project is not *worth* the time" (= *time is a valuable commodity*). The ability to access and utilize concepts of this type in discourse can be called, simply, *conceptual competence*.

What is the difference between *conceptual competence* and the two other types of competence identified by linguistics—namely, *linguistic* and *communicative competence*? *Linguistic competence* is knowledge of the language system in itself. It is comprised of various subcompetencies, the chief ones being *lexico-semantic*, *syntactic*, *morphological*, *phonological*, and *graphological* (writing):

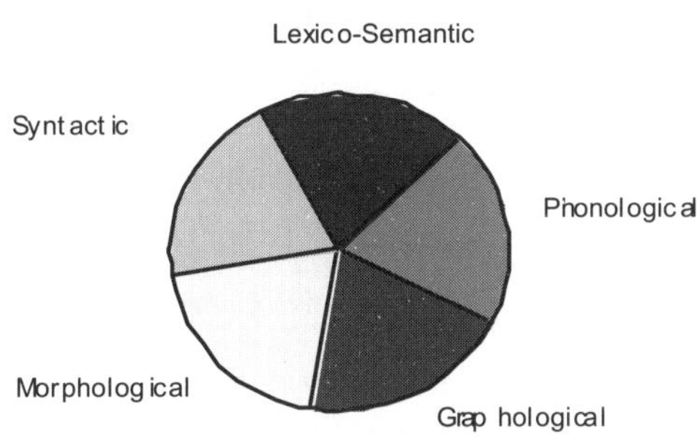

Figure 6. Linguistic Competence

Lexico-semantic competence involves knowing the meaning potential of language forms. It manifests itself in discourse as the ability to select forms and structures to match concepts appropriately. Syntactic competence involves the ability to organize forms for physical delivery in speech. This includes knowledge of basic phrase structure, of the ordering of the words within phrases, of agreement between structures (e.g. agreement of number and gender between subject and verb), of case structure (position and function of a word within a sentence), and of sentence types (e.g. negatives, interrogatives, etc.). Morphological competence involves the ability to recognize and inflect forms. Essentially, this entails knowing what constitutes a word and what units smaller than words (morphemes) convey meaning. Phonological competence is the ability to articulate sounds and utilize the sound system for expression in an appropriate fashion; and graphological competence is the ability to use the graphic system (alphabet characters, pictograms, etc.) to decipher and construct appropriate verbal texts.

Communicative competence is the ability to apply the language structures and categories to interactional and representational situations in an appropriate manner. Its main subcompetencies include *pragmatic*, *strategic*, and *stylistic* ones:

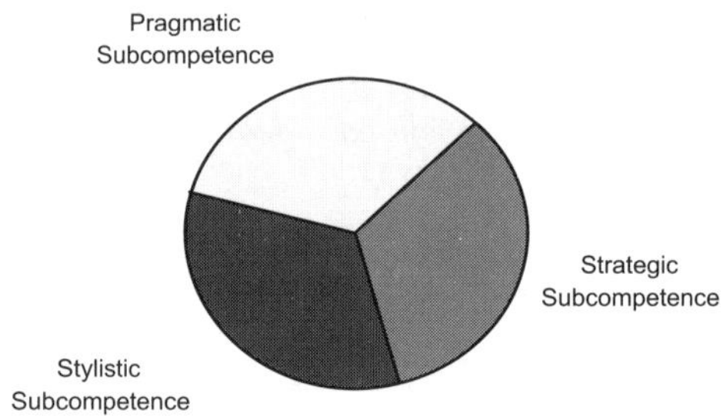

Figure 7. Communicative Competence

Pragmatic competence involves the ability to recognize and produce speech forms that fit a situation (saying hello, criticizing, etc.). Strategic competence is the ability to use language to carry out certain social interactions in a strategic way: e.g. cajoling, persuading, etc. And stylistic competence is knowledge of which register or style (formal, casual, etc.) is appropriate in a given situation or medium.

As Hymes (1971) showed, linguistic and communicative competencies are hardly autonomous psychological phenomena. The two are intrinsically intertwined. For example, to maintain the smooth flow of meaning in speech acts, it is necessary to know how to filter out repetitions in them. Consider, for instance, the following two accounts, which tell the same story in different ways:

1. Mary went to the store yesterday. Mary met a friend at the store. Mary and the friend greeted each other. Mary hadn't seen her friend in a long time.
2. Mary went to the store yesterday. She met a friend at the store. They greeted each other. Mary hadn't seen her in a long time.

The first one sounds stilted and odd, even though by itself, each sentence in it is well formed. The second version reads more like ordinary conversation because in English, as in other languages, repetition is discouraged in speech acts. For this reason, the language makes available several devices that allow for the same information to be rendered without the repetition.

Devices that refer back to some word or syntactic category are called *anaphoric*. In the text above, *she* refers back to *Mary*, *they* to *Mary and the friend*, and *her* to *her friend*. The counterpart of an anaphoric device is a *cataphoric* one. This is a word or particle used in anticipation of some other word. For example, in the sentence "Even if he denies it, I swear that Mark did it," the pronoun *he* refers ahead to *Mark*. Subject and object pronouns, locative particles, demonstratives, adverbs, and the like often function as anaphoric and cataphoric particles in conversations and written texts.

Another area in which the congruity between linguistic and communicative competence can be easily seen is in the pragmatic one. To greet a friend in Italian, it is necessary to use familiar forms (*Ciao, Alessandro* "Hi, Alexander"). Polite ones are required instead when greeting, say, a professor (*Buon giorno, professor Marchi* "Hello, Professor Marchi"). This kind of practical knowledge involves knowing *who* says *what* to *whom* in specific situations. many strides have been made in pragmatic study in the last four or five decades. The findings from that field are of obvious importance to both SLA and SLT.

As one last example of the interface between linguistic and communicative competencies, consider the speech function known as a *gambit*. A gambit is a word, phrase, or construction of some type used to open a conversation, to keep it going, to make it flow smoothly, to gain attention, to seek approval, etc. In English, for example, the following are gambits with three different functions:

1. Uh huh...ya...hmm...aha...
2. You agree with me, don't you?
3. May I ask you a question?

The grunt-like expression uttered in the first gambit acknowledges that one is listening to an interlocutor, especially on the phone. Total silence is not an appropriate gambit in English conversation, although it is in other languages. In Italian a different gambit is deployed for this function, namely a series of words such as, *sì...capisco...eh già...vero* ("yes...I understand...ah, yes... true"). The second gambit is known as a *tag question* (literally a question tagged on at the end of a sentence). It is designed in the sentence above as an agreement-seeking or consent-seeking strategy. The third gambit is, clearly, a conversation opener.

Conceptual competence is the ability to verbalize concepts so as to construct messages that have a culturally-appropriate structure, no matter what suitable syntactic or morphological form they assume. In a sense, conceptual competence can be considered to be the complex of ideas and images that come to mind when thinking of some abstraction and the kinds of words, syntactic structures, verb forms, etc. they suggest in a specific communicative context. It is intrinsically interconnected with referential and representational systems present in a culture, which overlap considerably with verbal semantic systems. In a phrase, a concept that is delivered in language in some specific way, or set of ways, will tend to be found in nonverbal systems in some form.

Conceptual competence consists of three main subcompetencies: *metaformal*, *reflexive*, and *associative*.

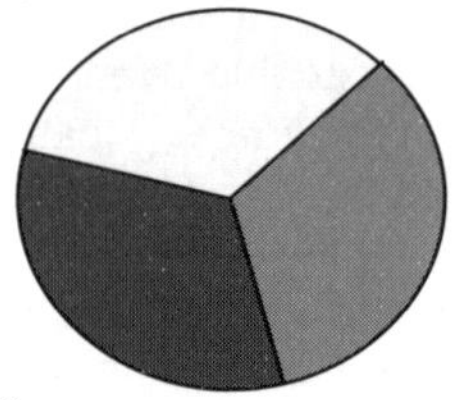

Figure 8. Conceptual Competence

Metaformal competence (as will be discussed below) is the ability to use the conceptual system of a language appropriately in speech. Reflexive competence involves the ability to transform concepts into language categories (syntactic, morphological, etc.). This is called *reflexive* because the view espoused here is that language encodes concepts by mirroring them in some physical or formal way. Finally, associative competence is knowledge of how concepts are interconnected to each other in cultural terms. Take, again, the example of *time* above. The *time is money* formula above can be defined as a *metaform* (as will be elaborated below). The linguistic choices made to encode this concept will, however, vary according to situation. In other words, they will be *reflexivized* differently:

As a verb:	I have *spent* too much time on that project.
As an adjective:	His time is *valuable*."
As a noun:	What's the *price* to be paid for her time?"

The ability to associate the *time is money* metaform to other metaforms (e.g. *time is a valuable commodity*) and to cultural perceptions of time is part of what constitutes *associative* competence. Conceptual competence is clearly interrelated with linguistic and communicative competence. This suggests that *proficiency* in a language is the ability to utilize all three competencies in an integrated, interdependent fashion—conceptual competence entails knowing what to say in a certain situation; communicative competence what that situation is and how to respond to it verbally; and linguistic competence how to realize the message in terms of the forms a language makes available.

The notion of conceptual competence makes it possible to pinpoint in a precise way the source of what has been called "conceptual errors" in the previous chapter. It also allows us to expand the conceptualization principle elaborated in the same chapter as follows:

The Conceptualization Principle Revised

> Student discourse invariably seems to lack the conceptual appropriateness that characterizes native speaker discourse. Students "speak" with the memorized formal and communicative structures of the SL, but they "think" in terms of their native conceptual system: i.e. students typically use SL words and communicative protocols as "carriers" of their own native language concepts. When the native and SL conceptual systems coincide, then student discourse is assessable as "natural;" when they do not, it manifests an asymmetry between language form and conceptual content. What student discourse often lacks, in other words, is conceptual fluency. This is clearly something that must be taken directly into account in SLT.

Neuroscientific Research on Metaphor

Before dealing with the implications of the above principle, it is necessary to step back and take a look at what the research on metaphor implies for any development of *Conceptual Fluency Theory* (CFT) in SLT. I start by considering the work on metaphor in neuroscience. Such work has established, first and foremost, that metaphor involves content-related functions in the RH and form-related ones in the LH, which are interconnected through complex neural networks. The evidence for this interhemispheric model came originally from the study of brain-damaged patients. In 1964, the psychologist Weinstein was among the first to conduct a clinical study demonstrating that patients with RH damage had lost the ability to comprehend and produce metaphors. This suggested an RH locus for metaphorical meanings. A study by Winner and Gardner (1977), a little more than a decade later, corroborated Weinstein's finding. The two researchers presented a series of utterances to various subjects asking them to select one of four pictures that best portrayed the meaning of the utterance. For the sentence *A heavy heart can really make a difference* the subjects were shown four pictures from which to choose:

1. a person crying (= metaphorical meaning);
2. a person staggering under the weight of a huge red heart (= literal meaning);
3. a 500-pound weight (= a representation emphasizing the adjective *heavy*);
4. a red heart (= a representation emphasizing the noun phrase *red heart*).

Of the subjects used in the study—aphasics (subjects with LH damage), patients with RH damage, and a normal control group—only the RH-damaged ones manifested consistent difficulties in identifying metaphorical meanings.

In the same year, Stachowiak, Huber, Poeck, and Kerschensteiner (1977) conducted a similar type of study and came to the same conclusion. These researchers read subjects stories and then asked them to pick from a set of five drawings the one which best described what happened to the main character of each one. One of the stories contained a metaphorical idiom was included. The groups tested were aphasics, RH patients, and normals. Like Winner and Gardner, the researchers found that, of the three groups, the RH patients were the ones who showed the greatest inability to detect the metaphorical idioms.

In the 1980s, the evidence in favor of an RH involvement in metaphor mounted. Hier and Kaplan (1980) found that RH patients exhibited deficits in explaining the meaning of proverbs. Wapner, Hamby, and Gardner (1981) discovered that RH patients tended to exhibit significant difficulties in deriving the metaphorical point of a story. Brownell, Potter, and Michelow (1984) and Brownell (1988) detected RH involvement in metaphor comprehension, but could not specify what neural regions of the RH were implicated. Using PET-scanning equipment Bottini et al. (1994) showed the right temporal lobe to be the most active one in metaphor. They also found that the right parietal lobe was active in some metaphorical tasks, whereas the corresponding lobe in the LH was not.

This line of research has definite implications for pedagogy, since it suggests that metaphor is a fundamental R-Mode feature. It has concrete implications, for instance, on how to structure novel input in the modal flow. These will be discussed below.

Conceptual Metaphor Theory

Interest in metaphor is ancient. It was Aristotle (384-322 BC), in fact, who coined the term *metaphor*—itself a metaphor (*meta* 'beyond' + *pherein* 'to carry')—pointing out that many abstract forms of knowledge are grounded in metaphorical reasoning. However, Aristotle also affirmed that, as knowledge-productive as it was, the most common function of metaphor was to spruce up literal ways of thinking and speaking. Remarkably, this latter assertion was the one that was embraced by most Western philosophers and linguists for two millennia. But nothing could have been farther from the truth. In 1977, the research team of Pollio, Barlow, Fine, and Pollio conducted an extensive investigation of common discourse texts and found them to be immersed in metaphorical reasoning. They concluded that speakers of English used on average 3,000 novel metaphors and 7,000 idioms per week. Obviously, they remarked, metaphor could hardly be considered an ornamental option to literal language.

Particularly influential in getting the study of metaphor onto the agenda of linguistics and psychology was George Lakoff and Mark Johnson's 1980 book *Metaphors We Live By*. The innovative claim of that book was that metaphor is the cornerstone of human cognition. First, Lakoff and Johnson asserted what Aristotle had claimed two millennia before, namely that there are two types of concepts—*concrete* and *abstract.* But the two scholars added a remarkable twist to this Aristotelian notion—namely that many *abstract concepts* are built up systematically from *concrete* ones through metaphorical reasoning. They designated such abstract concepts *conceptual metaphors*. For example, the expression "John is a gorilla" is an example of something more general, namely, *people are animals*. This is why we say that *John* or *Mary* or whoever is a *gorilla, snake, pig, puppy,* and so on. Each specific metaphor ("John is a gorilla;" "Mary is a snake," etc.) is not an isolated example of poetic fancy. Rather, it is an instantiation of a more general metaphorical idea—*people are animals*. Such ideas are what Lakoff and Johnson called *conceptual metaphors*:

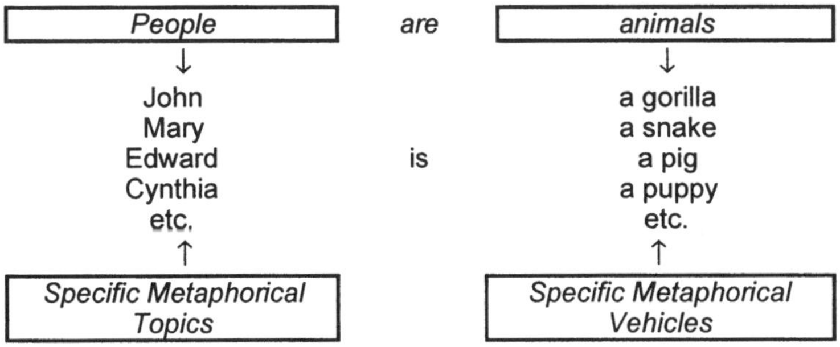

Figure 9. Conceptual Metaphor

Each of the two parts of the *conceptual metaphor* is called a *domain—people* is called the *target domain* because it is the abstract topic itself (the "target" of the conceptual metaphor); and *animals* is called the *source domain* because it encompasses the class of vehicles that delivers the metaphor (the "source" of the concept). An *abstract concept* of this type can now be defined simply as a "mapping" of one domain onto the other. The research on conceptual metaphors suggests that many abstract concepts are formed systematically through such mappings and that specific metaphors are traces to the target and source domains that a culture has established over time for the delivery of meanings in discourse and texts of all kinds. So, when we hear people talking, for instance, of *ideas* in terms of *geometrical figures and relations*—"Those ideas are *circular*," "I don't see the *point* of your idea," "Her ideas are *central* to the discussion," "Their ideas are *diametrically opposite*," etc.—we can now easily identify the two domains as *ideas* (= target domain) and *geometrical figures/relations* (= source domain) and, therefore, the conceptual metaphor as: *ideas are geometrical figures and relations*.

Conceptual metaphors pervade common discourse. A few examples will suffice to make this evident (Danesi 2000):

Happiness is up/Sadness is down

1. Today she's feeling *up*.
2. Generally she feels *down*.
3. His comment *boosted* my spirits.
4. My mood *sank* after she told me what happened.
5. His joke gave me a *lift*.

Health and life are up/Sickness and death are down

6. Everyone in my family is at the *peak* of health.

7. Unfortunately, my cousin *fell* ill.
8. My job is an *uphill* struggle.
9. Lazarus *rose* from the dead.
10. They're *sinking* fast.

Light is knowledge/Dark is ignorance

11. The whole class was *illuminated* by that professor.
12. I was left in the *dark* about what happened.
13. Her explanation is very *clear*.
14. Quantum theory is *obscure*.
15. His example *shed light* on several matters.

Theories are buildings

16. Hers is a *well-constructed* theory.
17. His theory too is on solid *ground*.
18. But that theory needs more *support*.
19. Otherwise the theory will *collapse* under criticism.
20. Alexander put together the *framework* of a very interesting theory.

Ideas and theories are plants

21. My professor's ideas have come to *fruition*.
22. That's a *budding* theory.
23. Plato's ideas have contemporary *offshoots*.
24. That idea has become a *branch* of mathematics.

Ideas are commodities

25. My friend certainly knows how to *package* his ideas.
26. However, that idea just won't *sell*.
27. There's no *market* for that idea.
28. That's a *worthless* idea.

We do not detect the presence of conceptual metaphors in such common expressions because of repeated usage. For instance, we no longer interpret the word *see* in sentences such as "I don't *see* what you mean," "Do you *see* what I'm saying?" in metaphorical terms, because its use in such expressions has become so familiar to us. But the association between the biological act of seeing outside the body with the imaginary act of seeing within the mind was originally the source of the conceptual metaphor *seeing is understanding/believing/thinking*, which now permeates common discourse, as can be seen in the examples given below which have become so common that we hardly ever stop to reflect upon how they are constructed conceptually:

29. There is more to this than *meets the eye.*
30. I have a different *point of view.*
31. It all depends on how you *look* at it.
32. I take a *dim view* of the whole matter.
33. I never *see eye to eye* on things with you.
34. You have a different *worldview* than I do.
35. Your ideas have given me great *insight* into life.

The next important point made by Lakoff and Johnson is that there are three general kinds of cognitive processes involved in metaphorical conceptualization. The first one involves mental *orientation*. This produces concepts that are derived from our physical experiences of *up vs. down, back vs. front, near vs. far*, etc. These experiences are converted into mental models of various abstractions that we sense may have something in common with the original physical experience. For example, the experience of *up vs. down* underlies such conceptual metaphors as:

36.	Happiness is up	= I'm feeling *up*.
37.	Sadness is down	= She's feeling *down* today.
38.	More is up	= My income *rose* (went up) last year.
39.	Less is down	= Her salary *went down*.

I would like to suggest that orientation is part of a larger sensorially-based cognitive strategy that may be called *sense-implication* (Sebeok and Danesi 2000). This refers to the tendency in abstract-concept formation of extrapolating sensory experiences that are felt intuitively to entail the concept in question. For instance, in conceptualizing *love* we typically extrapolate physiological experiences that we associate with romantic love in order to conceptualize it in some imagistically-meaningful way.

The following expressions, for instance, conjure up images that are not visually-orientated. Rather, they implicate other sensory modalities: (1) the *sound of thunder* (= auditory sense-implication); (2) the *feel of wet grass* (= tactile sense implication); (3) the *smell of fish* (= olfactory sense-implication); (4) the *taste of toothpaste* (= gustatory sense-implication); (5) the *sensation of being uncomfortably cold* (= bodily sense-implication); (6) the *sensation of extreme happiness* (= emotional sense-implication); etc.

The second type of conceptualization process, according to Lakoff and Johnson, involves *ontological* thinking. This produces conceptual metaphors in which activities, emotions, ideas, etc. are associated with entities, substances, objects, containers, etc.:

40.	time is a valuable commodity	= It's not *worth* my time.
41.	the mind is a container	= I'm *full* of memories.
42.	anger is fluid in a container	= My blood is *boiling*.

As a concrete example of how ontological thinking undergirds metaphorical conceptualization, consider the outline of an *impediment* or *obstacle*:

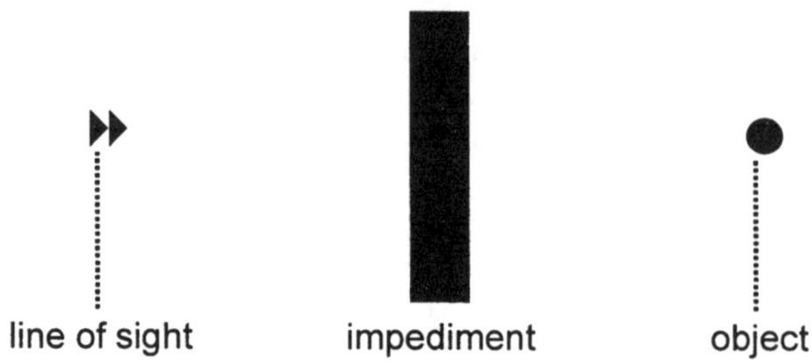

Figure 10. Impediment Schema

Several abstract scenarios are now imaginable in terms of this ontological scenario—one can *go around* the impediment, *go over* it, *under* it, *through* it, or *remove* it and *continue* on towards the object. On the other hand, the obstacle could successfully impede someone, so that one would *stop* at the impediment and *turn back*. These imaginary scenarios constitute the reason why we say such things as:

43. We *got through* that difficult time.
44. Jim felt better after he *got over* his cold.
45. You want to *steer clear* of financial debt.
46. With the bulk of the work *out of the way*, he was able to call it a day.
47. The rain *stopped us* from enjoying our picnic.
48. You cannot *go any further* with that idea; you'll just have to *turn back*.

The third type of process, Lakoff and Johnson suggest, is an elaboration of the other two. This produces *structural conceptual metaphors* that distend orientational and ontological concepts. A *structural conceptual metaphor* is a cognitive formula built from existing conceptual metaphors of an orientational or ontological nature: for example, the structural metaphor *time is money* is built from *time is a resource* and *time is a quantity*:

49. Time is a resource = The project was *consumed* much time.
50. Time is a quantity = *How much* time do you have?
51. Time is money = I *spent* too much time on that project.

In later work, Lakoff and Johnson referred to such mental processes as image *schemas* (Lakoff 1987, Johnson 1987). These are defined as largely unconscious mental images of recurrent shapes, actions, dimensions, objects, experiences, etc. that derive from perception and sensation. Image schemas are, clearly, the result of

R-Mode processes. They are so deeply rooted that we are hardly ever aware of their control over conceptualization. But they can always be conjured up easily. If a native-speaker of English were asked to explain an idiom such as *spill the beans*, he/she would not likely have a conscious image of beans and the action of spilling them. However, if that same person were to be asked the following questions—"Where were the beans before they were spilled?" "How big was the container?" "Was the spilling on purpose or accidental?" etc.—then he/she would no doubt start to visualize the appropriate schema—the beans are kept in a container; the container is about the size of the human head; etc.

To get a firmer sense of how conceptual metaphors shape common discourse, consider the *argument is war* concept. The target domain of *argument* is conceptualized in terms of *warlike activities* (the source domain), and thus in terms of *battles* that can be *won* or *lost*, of *positions* that can be *attacked* or *guarded*, of *ground* that can be *gained* or *lost*, of *lines of attack* that can be *abandoned* or *defended*, and so on. These warlike images are so embedded in our mind that we do not normally realize that they guide our perception of arguments. But they are nonetheless there, surfacing regularly in such common expressions as the following:

52. Your claims are *indefensible*.
53. You *attacked* all my *weak points*.
54. Your criticisms were *right on target*.
55. I *demolished* his argument.
56. I've never *won* an argument.
57. She *shot down* all my points.
58. If you use that *strategy*, I'll *wipe you out*.

The last relevant point made by Lakoff and Johnson in their truly fascinating book is that culture is built on metaphorical thinking, since conceptual metaphors coalesce into a system of meanings that holds together the entire network of associated meanings in the culture. This is accomplished by a kind of "higher-order" metaphorizing—i.e. as target domains are associated with many kinds of source domains (orientational, ontological, structural), the concepts they underlie become increasingly more complex, leading to what Lakoff and Johnson call *cultural* or *cognitive models*. To see what this means, consider the target domain of *ideas* again. The following three conceptual metaphors, among many others, deliver the meaning of this concept in the following three separate ways (again among many others):

Ideas are food

59. Those ideas left a *sour taste* in my mouth.
60. Its hard to *digest* all those ideas at once.
61. Even though he is a *voracious* reader; he can' t *chew* all those ideas
62. That teacher is always *spoon-feeding* her students.
63. That idea has *deep roots*.

Ideas are persons

64. Darwin is the *father* of modern biology.
65. Those medieval ideas continue to *live on* even today.
66. Cognitive linguistics is still in its *infancy.*
67. Maybe we should *resurrect* that ancient idea.
68. She *breathed* new life into that idea.

Ideas are fashion

69. Those scientists are the *avant-garde* of their field.
70. Those revolutionary ideas are no longer in *vogue.*
71. Semiotics has become truly *chic.*
72. That idea is an old *hat.*

Recall from other examples cited above that there are other ways of conceptualizing *ideas* in English—in terms of *buildings, plants, commodities, geometry, seeing*, etc. The constant juxtaposition of such conceptual formulas in common discourse produces, cumulatively, a *cognitive model* of ideas.

Before Lakoff and Johnson's trend-setting work, the study of metaphor fell within the field of *rhetoric*, where it was viewed as one of various *tropes*—i.e. figures of speech. But since the mid-1980s the practice has been to use the term *metaphor* to refer to the study of all figurative language and to consider the other tropes as particular kinds of metaphor. Within this new paradigm *personification*, for instance ("My cat speaks Chinese"), would be seen as a particular type of metaphor, one in which the target domain is an animal or inanimate object and the source domain a set of vehicles that are normally associated with human beings (the counterpart of the *people are animals* concept). Similarly, an *oxymoron* ("thunderous silence") would be considered to be a metaphor used to bring out contrast. However, there are two tropes that are regularly studied separately—*metonymy* and *irony*—because of their particular conceptual characteristics.

Metonymy is the use of an entity to refer to another that is related to it:

73. He likes *Bronte* (= the writings of Bronte).
74. My mom hates *nose rings* (= the fact that I am wearing them).
75. The *automobile* is destroying health (= the collection of automobiles).
76. How many *faces* are there in the audience (= people).
77. I bought a *Saturn* (= car named *Saturn*).
78. The *buses* are on strike (= bus drivers).
79. The *White House* was silent about the incident (= the president, the American government).

Synecdoche is a particular type of metonymy. It is the use of the part to represent the whole:

81. The *automobile* is destroying our health (= the collection of automobiles).
82. We need a couple of *strong bodies* for our teams (= strong people).
83. I've got a new *set of wheels* (= car).
84. We need *new blood* in this organization (= new people).

In parallelism with the notion of *conceptual metaphor*, *conceptual metonym* can thus be suggested as the cognitive form underlying such utterances (Sebeok and Danesi 2000). Here are some examples of conceptual metonyms:

The part stands for the whole

85. Get your *butt* over here!
86. The Blue Jays need a *stronger arm* in right field.
87. We don't hire *crew cuts*.

The producer stands for the product

88. I'll have a *Heineken*.
89. We bought a *Ford*.
90. He's got a *Rembrandt* in his office.

The object used stands for the user

91. My *piano* is sick today.
92. The *meat and potatoes* is a lousy tipper.
93. The *buses* are on strike.

The institution stands for the people behind it

94. *Shell* has raised its prices again.
95. The *Church* thinks that promiscuity is immoral.
96. I don't approve of *Washington's* actions.

The place stands for the institution

97. The *White House* isn't saying anything.
98. *Milan* is introducing new jackets this year.
99. *Wall Street* is in a panic.

The face is the person

100. He's just another *pretty face*.
101. There are an awful lot of *faces* in the audience.
102. We need some new *faces* around here.

It is interesting to note that metaphorical and metonymic concepts permeate many facets of cultural expression and behavior. The *face is the person* conceptual metonym, for instance, also crystallizes in the nonverbal domain, especially in the art of portraiture which emphasizes the face as equivalent to the character of the person. The conceptual metaphor *justice is blind* crops up not only in conversations, but also in pictorial representations. This is why there are statues of blindfolded women inside courtrooms to symbolize *justice*. The metaphorical expression *the scales of justice*, too, is evident in the sculptures of scales near or inside justice buildings. Similarly, the *love is a sweet taste* conceptual metaphor finds expression not only in discourse ("She's my *sweetheart*;" "I love my *honey*;" etc.), but in rituals of love-making in Western culture. This is why sweets are given to a loved one at St. Valentine's day, why matrimonial love is symbolized at a wedding ceremony by the eating of a cake, why lovers sweeten their breaths with candy before kissing, and so on.

Irony is the use of words to convey a contrary meaning—e.g. "I love being tortured." Ironic concepts produce meaning through contrast; i.e. by associating target domains (e.g. *torture, torment,* etc.) with incongruous source domains (*love, enjoyment*, etc.):

103. I love being tortured.
104. She loves getting hurt.
105. He enjoys torment.

Such instantiations are, in effect, manifestations of a single concept—*pain is understood by thinking of its opposites*. In affinity with the terms *conceptual metaphor* and *conceptual metonym*, such a concept can be called a *conceptual ironic form*. In effect, conceptual metaphors, metonyms, and ironic forms make up a large part of conceptual competence. In the realm of SLT, this type of competence has rarely, if ever, been taken directly into account. Yet, it is an intrinsic component of SLA, which simply must be integrated with linguistic and communicative competence.

Extending the Theory

Conceptual Metaphor Theory has been the target of extensive research since the publication of Lakoff and Johnson's book in 1980. Recently, Sebeok and Danesi (2000) suggest that the notions of *conceptual metaphor*, *conceptual metonym,* and *conceptual ironic form* be coalesced under one general rubric—which they call *metaform.* They define a metaform as a conceptual form that encodes meaning either by: (1) metaphorical association, (2) metonymic reference, or (3) ironic commentary. In this way, many abstract concepts can be treated as single forms, rather than as disparate conceptual phenomena. Metaforms, in fact, have the same semantic characteristics that single structures such as words do: i.e. they have:

- a *differentiative* meaning that set them apart from others (e.g. *people are animals* vs. *the face is the person*);

- an *associative* meaning, whereby connections are made and inferences drawn about them (if *time is money* then it is obvious that *money* plays a crucial role in the culture that has encoded this concept);
- a *preservative* meaning, whereby they become part of everyday representational activities and of communal beliefs (as we saw above with the nonverbal manifestations of metaforms);
- an *evaluative* meaning, whereby the can be discussed and tested further;
- a *perspectival* meaning, whereby their individual users become aware of the different perspectives of the world they entail.

Since the source domain of most metaforms encompasses concrete vehicles, it follows that the selection of one vehicle or another from a particular domain will produce connotative nuances. Take, for example the metaphorical statement "The professor is a *snake*," which is an instantiation of the metaform *people are animals*, as we saw above. The meaning of *snake* that this statement encodes, however, is not its concrete, denotative one. Rather, it encodes the culture-specific connotations perceived in snakes; namely "slyness," "danger," "slipperiness," etc. It is this complex of connotations that is implied in the utterance "The professor is a *snake*." Each different instantiation of this metaform changes the view we get of the topic: e.g. in "The professor is a *rat*," the *professor* is portrayed instead as someone "aggressive," "combative," "rude," etc.—a complex of connotations that are implicit in the new selected vehicle *rat*.

Once a metaform has been introduced into the system of concepts that makes up a culture, then it becomes itself a source for providing further descriptive detail to evaluations of, say, human personality, if such a need should arise. Thus, for instance, the specific utilization of *snake* as the vehicle can itself become a subdomain (made up of types of snakes), allowing one to zero in on specific details of the personality being described:

1. He's a *cobra*.
2. She's a *viper*.
3. Your friend is a *boa constrictor*.

Within each source domain, there are subdomains that provide the metaform-user with an array of connotative concepts that can be utilized to project subtle detail on to the description of a certain personality. The *people are animals* metaform is, in effect, a superordinate concept (previous chapter), because it refers to the general phenomenon of personality. The choice of specific metaphorical vehicles from the *animal* source domain—*snake, rat,* etc.—produces basic concepts, because the vehicular choices allow for reference to types of personalities. Finally, the selection of subtypes of *snakes*—*cobra*, *viper*, etc.—produces subordinate concepts that are needed for specialized purposes.

Once the first "layer" of metaforms in a language has been formed, then this layer itself becomes a new productive source domain for creating more abstract concepts. Layered associations among metaforms can thus be called *meta-*

metaforms. For example, in utterances such as the following the target domain of *ideas* is rendered by source domains that are themselves metaforms:

4. Where did you *think up* that idea?
5. I *thought over* carefully your ideas.
6. You should *think out* the whole problem before attempting to solve it.

The phrase *think up* elicits a mental image of upward movement, thus portraying the abstract referent as an object being extracted physically from a kind of mental terrain; *think over* evokes the image of scanning with the mind's eye; and *think out* elicits an image of extracting something so that it can be held up to the scrutiny of the mind's eye. These constructions allow speaks to locate and identify abstract ideas in relation to spatiotemporal contexts, although such contexts are purely imaginary. *Think up* is an instantiation of the meta-metaform *thinking is an upward motion + thoughts are objects*; *think over* is an instantiation of the meta-metaform *thinking is a scanning motion + thoughts are viewable objects*; and *think out* is an instantiation of the meta-metaform: *thinking is viewing + thoughts are substances*. For the sake of pedagogical argument, however, no distinction will be made henceforward between metaforms and meta-metaforms.

There is a third, even more abstract, layer of metaphorical association that can be called *metasymbolic.* This layer contains symbols that result from the association of metaforms to each other in different ways and in different layers. For example, a *rose* is a metasymbol for *love* in Western culture because it derives ultimately from the metaphorical layering of *love* to a *sweet smell*, to the color *red*, and to the notion that love grows like a *plant*.

The higher the density of layering, the more abstract and, thus, more culture-specific the concept. Metaforms such as the *thinking is seeing* one are relatively understandable across cultures: i.e. people from non-English-speaking cultures could easily figure out what the statements that instantiate this metaform mean if they were translated to them, because they connect concrete source domains—e.g. *seeing*—to abstractions—*thinking*—directly. *Meta-metaforms*, on the other hand, are more likely to be understood primarily in culture-specific ways, and are thus much harder to conceptualize and translate, because they connect already-existing metaforms to other metaforms. *Metasymbols* involve pure cultural knowledge. For example, in the art of *chiaroscuro*—the technique of using light and shade in painting, invented by the Italian baroque painter Michelangelo Merisi da Caravaggio (1573-1610), is a metasymbol, since it derives from the many metaphorical associations ascribed to *light* and *darkness*. It is also the conceptual source for the fact that *illumination* is emphasized by religions. So-called "visionary" or "revelatory" experiences are regularly portrayed in terms of dazzling sensations of light.

More often than not, metaforms and metasymbols are traces to a culture's historical past. A common expression such as *He has fallen from grace* would have been recognized instantly in a previous era as referring to the Adam and Eve story in the Bible. Today we continue to use it with only a dim awareness (if any) of its Biblical origins. Expressions that portray life as a journey—"I'm still a long *way* from my life goal;" "There is no *end* in sight to my agonizing life," etc.—are similarly rooted in Biblical narrative.

Revisiting the SLT Dilemma

The notion of conceptual competence is something that clearly needs to be addressed directly by SL teachers. In my view, one of the main reasons—if not *the* main one—why the SLT Dilemma has never really been resolved is because the notion of conceptual competence has never been taken into direct account by methodologists. Of course, before the work of Lakoff and Johnson, it is unlikely that methodologists could have anticipated that a large portion of native speaker knowledge involved metaforms. However, even in the post-Lakoff and Johnson era, very little has been done in developing a pedagogical response to their work on metaphor. The question is of course: How can conceptual competence be imparted?

In one anecdotal study I conducted during the 1998 academic year, the following passage was given to several intermediate classes of SL students of Italian at the University if Toronto. They were asked to translate it into Italian:

> Jack is a real cool cat. He never blows his stack and hardly ever flies off the handle. What's more, he knows how to get away with things. Of course, he is getting on, too. His hair is pepper and salt, but he knows how to make up for lost time by taking it easy. He gets up early, works out, and turns in early.

This passage is, clearly, rich in metaforms and thus poses a truly difficult translation task. Needless to say, all the students found it, initially, difficult to "conceptualize" how the passage would be rendered in Italian. However, with the help of the instructor and the guided use of reference materials (dictionaries, phrase books), the students were gradually able to translate it in ways that reflected appropriate Italian versions to various degrees of fidelity, as native speakers confirmed subsequently by reading and assessing the translations.

One student made the following analogies that allowed her to reconfigure the text and, thus, reconceptualize in a culturally-appropriate Italian manner. In this case, the analogies rendered the text much more literal, yet still appropriate conceptually. The word "literal" is used in a relative sense, because most of the words chosen by the student are, in effect, either metaphors or have metaphorical derivations. For example, the word *cavarsela*, which she chose to render the concept of "to get away with something" is formed with the verb *cavare*. which means "to dig out, to take out/off," thus having a latent metaphorical meaning. As such, it is an instantiation of the conceptual metaphor *digging out is avoiding some consequence*. The image schemas in the two languages, although different, spring clearly from a similar kind of metaphorical inference, since the relevant conceptual metaphor in English is *getting away is avoiding some consequence*. Indeed, it is in making such explicit cultural comparisons that students will be in a better position to gain conceptual competence and, thus, be able to construct sentences and discourses that are native-like in their overall semantic and referential structure:

Table 5. Analogies between English and Italian Expressions

English	Italian
to be a (real) cool cat	*essere una persona molto calma*
to blow one's stack	*perdere l'auto-controllo, arrabbiarsi*
to fly off the handle	*arrabbiarsi fortemente*
what's more	*per di più*
to get away with something	*cavarsela*
of course	*certo, naturalmente*
to be getting on	*invecchiarsi*
pepper and salt	*capelli un po' grigi*
to make up for something	*riprendere, riacquistare, rifare*
lost time	*tempo perduto*
to take it easy	*stare calmo, non preoccuparsi*
to get up	*alzarsi dal letto*
to work out	*fare esercizio, fare ginnastica*
to turn in	*andare a dormire la sera*

Each substitution entailed a different *reflexivization*. This led her to produce several drafts that were edited for grammar and vocabulary. The end result was a composition that delivered the same message as the English one, but in conceptually-appropriate Italian, albeit much more denotative in its conceptual focus.

A follow-up study was designed to determine if conceptual knowledge could be used explicitly, not only in translating difficult passages, but also in teaching students to write conceptually-appropriate texts. During the 2000-2001 academic year, four high schools in the city of Toronto where Italian was taught in grade 11 were chosen for the study. The teachers in two of the schools were asked to use a similar approach to the one above to teach writing. The main components of this approach were as follows:

- Students were told to write down their ideas in their NL in any fashion they desired: i.e. they were told to indicate *what* they wanted to say in a composition.
- They were then instructed to connect the ideas among themselves with appropriate NL words and structures.
- Their NL "conceptual model" was then compared to corresponding texts composed in the SL (selected or written by the teacher).
- The students were then required to list the SL conceptual devices used in such texts, comparing them to those they used themselves in preparing their NL conceptual model, with the help of appropriate reference materials and the teacher.
- The students were then allowed to write a draft copy of the composition in the SL.
- The draft was then examined by the teacher for its conceptual correctness. All problems were discussed in terms of conceptualization—i.e. what words or structures delivered the concepts appropriately.

- When it was determined that the composition was conceptually appropriate, the student and teacher working together edited it for language and style.

The other two classes constituted a control group—i.e. one not taught according to the above format. The students wrote 123 compositions altogether. They were then given to native-speakers of Italian to assess them for their conceptual appropriateness. Except for a few cases, the speakers generally found the compositions written by the experimental classes to be superior to the compositions that the other students wrote. The speakers were asked to assign letter grades to the compositions— A, B, C, or D. The average obtained by the conceptually-trained students was A, whereas that of the control group was C. Although the study in no way constitutes a controlled experiment, it nevertheless provided a positive indication that conceptual competence can be imparted in a classroom situation.

Conceptual Systems in Contact

The above discussion raises several key issues with regard to classroom SLT. The main one is that differences between the NL and SL conceptual systems will have to be taken directly into account in the formulation of any effective pedagogical response to the SLT Dilemma. Our conceptual systems are culturally transmitted to us, through language, through our use and understanding of the language, and through other representational activities to which we are exposed in a culture (movies, TV programs, novels, newspapers, etc.). However, we are largely unaware that they even exist and do not question their validity.

Therefore, when students learn a new language, not only are two "language systems" in contact—the native and second ones, but also two "conceptual systems." The relevant systems can be symbolized as follows:

L1	= the learner's native language
CS1	= the learner's native conceptual system
L2	= the target language
CS2	= the conceptual system of the target culture

Now, the task of gaining proficiency in the SL can be formulated as follows:

SL Proficiency

SL proficiency involves the ability to express oneself in the L2 while utilizing the CS2, rather than using the L2, but relying primarily on the CS1.

Knowledge of the CS2 is not simply a question of familiarity with unique cultural concepts, such as the Spanish bullfight, the Tibetan practice of sand painting, or the Italian *passeggiata*. Rather, to be *conceptually fluent* is to be able to participate in a target culture's system of concepts, concrete and abstract. During the earliest phases of SLA, learners unconsciously rely on their CS1 to decipher novel input. They also express themselves largely through a process of conceptual translation, relying on the CS1 to direct the choice of L2 structures. Gradually, and with greater mastery of the L2, the students gain higher and higher levels of proficiency only if they have learned to access the CS2 directly. It is more the CS1 that will influence the acquisition of the L2, than the L1 considered as a system of structures.

It is entirely possible that even during the earliest stages learners will produce grammatically and conceptually native-like utterances, even though they are relying on the CS1. The reason for this is positive conceptual transfer, whereby L2 expressions result as native-like because the CS1 and CS2 overlap in a specific domain. Clearly, the individual concepts shared by two conceptual systems in contact will vary, depending on the particular languages and cultures in question. It is safe to assume, however, that there will indeed be overlap, and that this is a possible source of positive conceptual transfer for learners.

A Conceptually-Based CA

The above discussion constitutes an argument in favor of a conceptually-based CA. This would allow the teacher to determine how abstract concepts are formed in the L2 and how they are understood. Related to this is the question of determining which abstractions are more or less "productive" in a culture, i.e. are used to a greater or lesser degree for representational, ritualistic, and communicative purposes and activities. Is the concept of *love* more or less productive than, say, *justice* in a specific culture? That is to say, does the concept of *love* surface more often in texts, in discourse, and in social rituals than does the concept of *justice*? Is there a way of determining, or even "measuring," the relative productivity of these two concepts? Clearly, seeking answers to questions such as these is potentially important on several counts, not the least of which is determining if certain concepts are important to SLA.

To grasp what a conceptually-based CA might entail, consider the use of *avere* ("to have"), *fare* ("to do, make"), and *essere* ("to be") in expressions the involve the states of "coldness" and "hotness" in Italian (the L2) and English (the L1):

1.	*Fa freddo/caldo fuori.*	=	It is cold/hot outside.
2.	*Lui ha freddo/caldo.*	=	He is cold/hot.
3.	*Il caffè è freddo/caldo.*	=	The coffee is cold/hot.

The different verbal selections, together with the underlying conceptual systems that occasioned them can be shown in diagram form below, which constitutes, in effect, a CA of the two systems in question (CS1 = English, CS2 = Italian) in view of the differential verbal selections involved in the L1 (English) and the L2 (Italian):

L1	L2
It *is* cold/hot outside.	*Fa* freddo/caldo fuori.
↕	↕
CS1 *coldness/hotness is a physical state*	CS2 *coldness/hotness is an entity contained by Nature*
L1 He *is* cold/hot.	L2 Lui *ha* freddo/caldo.
↕	↕
CS1 *coldness/hotness is a physical state*	CS2 *coldness/hotness is an entity contained by someone*
L1 The coffee *is* cold/hot.	L2 Il caffè è freddo/caldo.
↕	↕

CS1 = CS2
coldness/hotness is a physical state

Figure 11. Conceptual Systems in Contact

In Italian, the verb *fare* is used with respect to a weather situation—*fa freddo* (literally) "it makes cold," *fa caldo* (literally) "it makes hot." The physical state of "coldness" or "hotness" is conveyed instead by the verb *essere* when referring to objects (*è freddo* "it is cold," *è caldo* "it is hot") and by *avere* "to have" when referring to people (*ha freddo* "he/she is cold", *ha caldo* "he/she is hot"). The use of one verb or the other—*fare, essere,* or *avere*—is clearly motivated by an underlying metaformal conceptualization of bodies, objects, and the environment as *containers* and the states of "coldness" and "hotness" as *entities*. The *container* and *entity* schemas are the sources of the differential verbal selections. If the *container* is the environment, then the *entities* ("coldness" and "hotness") are *made* by Nature *(fa freddo, fa caldo)*; if it is a human being, then the individual's body *has* them *(ha freddo, ha caldo)*; and if it is an object, then the object *is* their container *(è freddo, è caldo)*. No such conceptual distinctions are required by the English CS1.

This type of CA can thus be employed to explain an error of the type **Lui è freddo*, which can be traced to a negative transfer originating in the CS1, as would **Il caffè ha freddo.* This type of analysis has, clearly, a concrete pedagogical implication: When teaching about "coldness" and "hotness" in Italian it is essential to relate the selection of the verbs to the *container* schema. In this way, the CS2 will be brought directly into pedagogical account.

Interest in incorporating such a view of CA into mainstream SLT has been minimal. Only one movement, called the *Contrastive Rhetoric Movement*, that took root in 1966 (Kaplan 1966), can be seen to have some of the same pedagogical interests discussed in this chapter. The key finding of this movement (Kaplan 1978, Kroll 1990, Leki 1991, Connor 1996, Chesterman 1998) is that a large portion of negative transfer occurs on a rhetorical conceptual level rather than on purely a lexical or syntactic level. Typically, unless they have learned the appropriate domains of the CS2, the students' attempts at SL discourse will "violate the expectations of the native reader" (Kaplan 1966: 4). The claim of the movement is that conceptual competence—as it has been called here—is as teachable as linguistic or communicative competence. A contrastive rhetoric methodologist, Leki (1991), recounts an anecdote of Fan Shen, a Chinese student who initially had trouble with her writing in English and then realized that it was more than just a question of stylistics, but rather a question of self-expression that was deeply rooted in her personality as it had developed in terms of her Chinese CS1. When her ESL teacher suggested that she "be herself" when writing something, Shen disagreed. Indeed, she correctly pointed out that in order to express herself in the L1, she needed to develop an "English Self," rooted in the CS2.

In developing a fully functional CA based on conceptual analysis, the notion of productivity arises: i.e. how productive is one concept in the CS1 vis-à-vis the CS2? The appropriate question would be: How many source domains are used, in a regular fashion, to deliver an abstraction such as *thinking* in the L2 with respect to the L1? How does the productivity of the concept compare with that of other abstract concepts? Is the concept more or less productive than it is in the native language? And, if so, does it lead to differential representational activities?

With a small group of research assistants at the University of Toronto, a pilot project was initiated in early 2000 to seek initial answers to a few of such questions. The team gathered data derived from a variety of English and Italian written and oral texts (newspapers, magazines, popular books, etc., recordings of radio and television programs). From the data, a list of conceptual metaphors related to two abstractions—*ideas* and *love*—was compiled. This was achieved simply by collecting statements related to the two concepts. From the list, the relevant source domains could be easily distinguished and categorized. Thus, for example, it was found that in English *ideas* (and their incorporation in such activities and events as laws, performances, lectures, etc.) was rendered by such source domains as *moving things, light and darkness, buildings, plants, commodities, vision, geometry, food, people, fashion,* among others.

The research team found, altogether (on the basis of nearly 100 written and oral texts), a total number of 89 source domains used to deliver the concept of *ideas* (or *thinking*). This can be called its *Productivity Index* (PI = 89). Given the number of texts used, by regular statistical inferencing, it can be considered to be a reliable metric for this specific concept: i.e. there is no reason to believe that a compilation of similar data would yield significantly different results (within regular margins of statistical error). Some source domains were enlisted more frequently than others. This could, of course, be a matter of style (some types of texts tend to manifest the utilization of certain source domains more than others), or a true index of productivity within the target domain. The pilot project did not control for this aspect of conceptual productivity (henceforward) CP. It emerged as a consequence of the study and, thus, is an issue that will have to be investigated in future work on CP. For the present purposes, the PI can be defined, simply, as a relative quantitative indication of the productivity of a concept, given a specific sample of data.

The PI of *thinking* was then compared to the PI of *love* (using the same database). The latter manifested itself through the medium of such source domains as *physics* ("There were *sparks* between the two actors"), *health and disease* ("The roles focused on the *sick* relationship between them"), *insane symptoms* ("He's *gone mad* over her"), *magic* ("She has *bewitched* her lover"), among others. The PI for *love* was found to be 36. This suggests that *love* is a less productive concept than *thinking* in English. To compare the two, the notion of *Relative Productivity Index* (RPI) was used. This is defined, simply, as the quotient that emerges when the lower PI is divided into the higher one. In the data collected, this turns out to be 2.47 (RPI = 2.47). This means, in effect, that there are 2.47 more source domains used for delivering *thinking* than there are for delivering *love* in English.

What does this imply? It suggests, arguably, that in English culture, *thinking* is a concept that is given much more representational salience, so to speak, than is *love*. This does not mean that the latter is not important, but, simply that there are fewer ways to conceptualize it in everyday cultural groupthink. It is left for future work to investigate whether differential RPIs lead to differences in cultural forms of expression.

The notion of CP can also be used to compare conceptual systems cross-culturally in a specific way. Knowledge of some of the source domains above—*food, people,* and *clothing*—is relatively independent of culture. However, there are some source domains that appear to be are dependent upon cultural knowledge. A comparative analysis will not only identify these, but also allow us to compare the RPI of certain concepts cross-culturally.

In the Italian data, it was found that most of the source domains used to deliver the concept of *thinking* were identical (even though their morphological and syntactic manifestations varied predictably). For example, *geometrical figures* ("Their ideas are *parallel*"), *vision* ("We couldn't *see* what he meant"), *food* ("Those ideas are hard to *swallow*"), etc. were frequent in the Italian data. More than completely identical source domains, however, the researcher team found that the nature of the source domain, in most cases, was slightly different. For example, rather than *plants* (e.g. "That idea has many *ramifications*), which also exists in Italian, the notion of *fertility* emerged as more productive in delivering the target domain (e.g. "Quella politica è veramente *arida*" = "That policy is truly *arid*"), as did *meteorological events* ("Le sue sono idee *tempestose*" = "His ideas are tempestuous;" "*Piovono* nuove idee in quell'università" = "New ideas are *raining* on that university") and *weight* ("Una delle sue idee è, comunque, un'idea assai *leggera*" = "One of his ideas is rather *light*"), among others. Overall, the Italian PI came to 123. The RPI between Italian and English in this domain was, therefore, 1.38 (which means that the Italian data showed 1.38 more source domains than the English data in the delivery of *ideas*). Needless to say, this is just an initial figure and would have to be tested again with other kinds of data. But, inferentially-speaking, there is no reason to believe that similar results would not emerge. The PI for *love* in Italian came to 99. Within Italian, this showed that the RPI (= 1.24) between the two target concepts of *thinking* and *love* is probably statistically irrelevant. However, it is significant when the PIs for *love* in English and Italian are compared (RPI = 2.75). Thus, there were almost three times as many source domains used to verbalize and represent *love* in the Italian data than there were in the English data.

When one talks about *ideas* or *love,* it is tantamount to "source-domain navigation," by which one passes (mentally) from *food* to *plants,* to *buildings,* etc. producing stretches of discourse such as: "I cannot quite *swallow* that new theory, even though it is claimed to have many *ramifications*, and can lead to a new *framework* of understanding, etc." The notion of CP is, arguably, a predictor of what domains are more likely to be involved in the navigation and which concepts are likely to be more or less productive during it.

Related to the notion of PI is *Source Domain Productivity* (SDP). This provides, simply, a comparative measure of the vehicles utilized within source domains: e.g. the *seeing* source domain above is highly productive in English and Italian for the delivery of *thinking*; however, the *moving things* one is rather limited in both languages, since very few vehicles in the domain are selected to deliver the concept. In effect, the SDP of the former is higher than that of the latter in both languages: in English it is 25 and 5, in Italian 29 and 12 for *seeing* and *moving things* respectively. Once again, this suggests that some metaphors are more frequent in discourse, representation, etc. than are others. In effect, within each source domain, there are sub-domains that provide the concept-user with an array of specific vehicles that can be utilized to provide subtle detail to some concept. The higher the SDP, the more likely the utilization of that source domain.

Concepts can also be compared in terms of source domains. If two concepts use identical source domains (in part or in whole), then they would have an identical PI. For example, *friendship* and *love* tend to be delivered in terms of identical (or similar) source domains:

> depth
>
> Theirs is a *profound* friendship/Theirs is a *profound* love.
>
> duration
>
> Theirs was a *brief* friendship/ Theirs was a *brief* love affair.

directionality

Their friendship is *continuing on*/ Their love affair is *continuing on.*

taste

Theirs is a *sweet* friendship/Their love is *sweet.*

etc.

In sum, the findings of the pilot project suggest one possible course for future work in the domain of conceptually-based CA. The relative indexes discussed provide, overall, a specific picture of conceptual productivity which, in turn, has implications for studying discourse and cultural representation generally. Cross-culturally, PIs, RPIs, and SDPs provide a basis upon which to compare concepts and derive whatever implications one might seek from the comparisons. Methodologically, all that is required is collecting sufficient textual data and sifting from it the relevant abstract concepts so as to quantify the source domains utilized. Needless to say, while metaphor is the conceptual glue that holds cultural meaning systems together, it is also the source of innovation in such systems. This is why novel metaphors are being created all the time. This means that PIs, RPIs, and SDPs will be constantly in flux.

Practical Implications

Previous research on conceptual competence (Danesi 1992, 1993c, Russo 1997) suggests that typical classroom learners show virtually no traces of conceptual fluency (CF), even after several years of study. The reason for this is not that they are incapable of learning the CS2, but rather that they have never been exposed to it in systematic ways. At the present time there seems to be very little in SL methodology that takes conceptual competence into account in any orderly fashion.

This does not imply a radical change in instruction. Rather, it entails a refocusing of traditional practices and techniques. During a graduate summer course I gave to high school teachers of Italian at Middlebury College in the summer of 1996, I found that conceptual competence was a notion that could easily be converted into practice. The student-teachers were taught the basic implications derived from the conceptualization principle and then asked to prepare a unit on either *love* or *birthdays* (Danesi 2000).

The first thing that they were required to do was to write dialogues. One student-teacher wrote a dialogue on birthdays that was structured conceptually by the metaform *age is a quantity.* This underlies expressions in native-speaker discourse such as the following:

> *Li porti bene gli anni* (literally "You carry your years well").
>
> *Gli anni incominciano a pesare sulle mie spalle* (literally "The years are beginning to weigh on my shoulders").

Quanti anni hai? Ne ho 22 (literally "How many years do you have? I have 22 of them").

The dialogue was then evaluated by three native speakers (professors from Italy visiting Middlebury College that summer) who found it to be "authentic" when compared to those found typically in textbooks. Here is an excerpt from her dialogue:

Role A: *Ciao, Marco, Ho sentito che oggi compi gli anni?*
("Hi Mark, I heard it's your birthday today").

Role B: *Eh, già.*
("That's right").

Role A: *Quanti ne hai?*
("How old are you?").

Role B: *Troppi! Oggi ne faccio 35.*
("Much too old. I'm 35 years old today").

Role A: *Ma, li porti veramente bene.*
("You wouldn't be able to tell").

The student-teachers were then asked to prepare explanatory, grammatical, and activity materials, following up on their dialogue-writing exercise. The quality of their work in this domain of pedagogy also demonstrated the facility with which conceptually appropriate practical material can be devised. The student-teacher who composed the above dialogue explained the verbs *portare* and *compiere*, the noun *anni*, and the particle *ne* as L2 structures tied to the CS2. Then, she introduced expressions such as *Ho due anni più/meno di te* ("I am two years older/younger than you"), expanding upon the novel input of the unit. Finally, she prepared conceptually-focused exercises, such as the following:

Quanti anni hanno i tuoi amici e come li portano?
("How old are your friends, and how do they look for their age?")

Chi ha più/meno anni di te?
("Who is older/younger than you?")

Quanti ne hanno?
("How old are they?")

She also prepared fill-ins, completions, multiple choices, etc. to bring out the conceptual structure of the *age is a quantity* metaform. This mechanical practice component was followed by typical role-playing and textual analysis activities. Without going here into details, suffice it to say that the Middlebury experiment showed that the notion of conceptual competence is as teachable and usable in the creation of units as is any other pedagogical notion. By simply structuring designated units of study around metaforms and metasymbols and then by presenting the appropriate grammar and communication patterns of the language as *reflexivizations* of these, the result seems to be a pedagogical product that is as usable as is any other kind of pedagogical artifact. Clearly, the modal flow principle is operative here since the conceptual focus of an exercise is R-Mode in its orientation—focusing on content—flowing through L-Mode components (whereby concepts are matched to structures), and finally resulting in an intermodal control of the thematic area.

Suggestions exist in the relevant pedagogical literature that fit in nicely with the idea of *conceptual fluency* (CF). Masella and Portner (1981), for instance, explore ways in which Italian terms referring to the human body can be extended to cover large stretches of the conceptual territory charted by these terms. Shibles (1989) shows how easily metaphorical vehicles for emotion in German can be compared to English ones for pedagogical purposes in ways that are very similar to the ones suggested here. Nuessel and Cicogna (1993) illustrate how metaphorical reasoning can be used as the basis of teaching new material.

Consider, as a case-in-point, the topic of sports in Italian. The crucial first step in a conceptually-based approach is to identify the main source domains that allow native speakers to deliver this concept in discourse. Here are seven of them (note that these overlap with English conceptual domains):

Table 6. Conceptualizing Sports in Italian

Conceptual Domain	Examples of actual discourse
fortune	Quella squadra è *fortunata* ("That team is fortunate") La loro vincita era *imprevedibile* ("Their victory was unpredictable")
war	Quella squadra è stata *sconfitta* ("That team was defeated") Quella squadra ha un buon *attacco* ("That team has a good attack) Quella partita è stata una *battaglia* ("That game was a battle")
board game	Che bella *mossa*! ("What a great move!") Quella squadra sa *regolare* il gioco ("That team knows how to regulate the game")
economics	Quella squadra ha *incassato* dei bei gol ("That team has cashed in on several beautiful goals") Quella squadra ha *pagato* il gol ("That team paid for the goal").
food	Quella squadra ha una *fame* di vincere ("That team is hungry for wins") Loro sono *digiuni* di vittorie ("They are on a diet of victories")
thought system	Hanno un'ottima *filosofia* di gioco ("They have an excellent playing philosophy") Quella squadra ha acquisito una *mentalità* vincente ("That team has developed a winning mentality")

After this initial analysis, the teacher can then resort to straightforward traditional pedagogy: i.e. the teacher may want to do such things as:

- prepare dialogical material that exemplifies the concepts;
- expose the students to actual sports broadcasts, highlighting how these concepts are employed;
- prepare exercise and activity material, whereby the students must identify the domains and explain them;
- require the students to write their own sportscast using the above analysis as a framework;

  etc.

But how would grammar be taught in such an instructional approach? As a concrete example of how to relate grammar to underlying conceptual structure consider the following sentences:

1. I have been living here *since* 1980.
2. I have known Lucy *since* November.
3. I have not been able to sleep *since* Monday.
4. I have been living here *for* 23 years.
5. I have known Lucy *for* nine months.
6. I have not been able to sleep *for* five days.

An analysis of the complements that follow *since* and *for* reveals that those that follow the former are "points in time," i.e. they are complements that reflect a metaformal conceptualization of *time* as *a "point" on a "line"* which shows specific years, months, etc.: "1980," "November," "Monday." Complements that follow *for*, on the other hand, reflect a conception of *time* as *a quantity*: "23 years," "nine months," "five days." These two metaforms—*time is a point on a line* and *time is a quantity*—can now be seen to have a specific effect at the level of syntax by motivating a grammatical dichotomy—complements introduced by *since* are reflexes of *time is a point on a line*; those introduced by *for* are reflexes of *time is a quantity*. This is, in fact, the kind of rule of grammar that allows the teacher to relate how two specific domains of conceptualization have worked their way into the grammatical system. In a word, this rule stipulates how a grammatical dichotomy *reflexivizes* a conceptual dichotomy.

In Italian, on the other hand, this rule does not exist—*da* is always used: *Vivo qui dal 1980*; *Vivo qui da ventitrè anni*, and so on. Students of Italian will be in a better position to avoid making typical errors such as **Vivo qui per ventitrè anni*, when they learn to conceptualize *time* in Italian appropriately, grasping the conceptual differences between "time in English" and "time in Italian." Explaining the phenomenon of *da* in such cases in any other way (e.g. in purely grammatical or lexical terms) continues to be a source of conceptual errors. This was borne out, albeit only tentatively, by a classroom study conducted at the Ontario Institute for Studies in Education in 1998. Fourteen student-teachers of Italian were divided into two equal groups: group A was instructed to teach *da* in time expressions according to traditional textbook explanations (which focus typically on the verbal tense); group B was instructed to teach it conceptually in the manner described above. The experiment took place during a regularly-scheduled practice-teaching session. At the end of the session, which lasted 3 weeks, the students taught by the student-teachers in each classroom were given a simple written cloze test, consisting of a paragraph in which 15 prepositions were missing. Of the 15 slots 6 had to be filled in with *da* reflecting time concepts. The other slots were there as distracters. There were 79 students taught by group A student-teachers—*A-taught* students—and 69 by group B student-teachers—*B-taught* students. Only 26 of the 79 A-taught students, or 32.9%, filled in the 6 slots with the correct preposition; on the other hand, 62 of the 69 B-taught students, or 89.9%, filled in the 6 slots correctly. The same experiment was repeated the year after with a different group of teachers and different classrooms. The results were the same—the students taught with a conceptual focus scored 92.3%; the others scored 38.5%.

For the sake of historical accuracy, it should be mentioned that the so-called *notional-functional* theorists championed an early version of the conceptualization principle in the early 1970s (e.g. Van Ek 1975, Wilkins 1976). Throughout that decade their syllabus was greeted with widespread enthusiasm throughout Europe and America. But it was largely abandoned by the mid-1980s because, in my view, the "notions" they elaborated were not connected to the CS2 in any systematic way. The teacher was simply given a typology of notions with verbal illustrations. A conceptually-based CA, as illustrated in this chapter, was never envisaged by the functional-notional methodologists. This is not to berate the excellent work done by them. The research on metaphor that has now become so widely known was not available to them at the time.

The important question for future work on developing a "conceptual syllabus" would thus seem to be: (1) To what extent do the conceptual systems of the native and target cultures overlap and contrast? (2) What kinds of conceptual interferences come from the student's CS1 (interconceptual interference)? (3) How much conceptual interference is generated by the target language itself (intraconceptual interference)? and (4) If concepts are to be placed at the core of language courses and syllabi, on what basis should they be selected and sequenced? The latter question is especially critical. In my view, the conceptual syllabus should be integrated with grammatical and communicative syllabi. As illustrated above, units in a course of study, for instance, could be planned around topics such as "time," "love," "health."

Not all domains of SLA are tied to the conceptual system, as it has been defined here. The interlanguage studies have amply documented error phenomena that are purely grammatical, communicative, etc. We should, of course, continue to assess the role played by linguistic and communicative competencies in the overall process of classroom SLA. However, if we are truly to "fine tune the brain" for SLA, then the notion of conceptual competence must be taken into account.

CHAPTER 5
ACTIVATING THE BRAIN IN THE CLASSROOM

We teachers can only help the work going on, as servants wait upon a master.

Maria Montessori (1870-1952)

Introduction

Since the Reform Movement, research on why it is so difficult to learn a SL in a classroom situation and what can be done to make it less of a struggle allowed teachers to make great strides in tackling the SLT Dilemma in the twentieth century. As we saw in the opening chapter, the initial "scientific" response to the Dilemma was the DM, which the reformers believed would facilitate the SLA process on its own, regardless of who was doing the teaching. The DM did not last. But teachers did not, as a consequence, abandon the method notion. On the contrary, they seemed to believe that sooner or later they would find the "right theoretical ingredients" to help them construct the "method to end all methods." The ALM was thought to be *that* method. But it too did not last. So, by the late 1960s it became obvious that something other than the "method response" to the SLT Dilemma was needed.

Of all the post-method "trends," the foray into the neurosciences has, in my view, produced some of the more interesting insights for tackling the SLT Dilemma. The principles elaborated in the previous two chapters are four such insights. The *modal flow* and *modal focusing* principles suggest that the two fundamental modes of learning—the experiential R-Mode and the analytical L-Mode—should operate at times in sequence, at others in parallel, and in a few instances in isolation. Moreover, they suggest that the flow of learning novel material cannot be hurried or circumvented. The contextualization principle implies that new language forms and concepts must be accompanied by contextual information in both the R-Mode and L-Mode phases of learning to enhance SLA. Finally, the conceptualization principle suggests that students need to become conceptually fluent—i.e. to gain control over the SL conceptual system—in order to achieve true proficiency. These four principles, when taken together, imply that the individual teacher will have to play a more critical role in the classroom than the traditional methods and the learner-centered approaches have calculated in the past. It is the teacher who will have to decide when the modal flow should be activated and when some phase can be "entered or exited," by becoming a keen observer of students, rather than relying primarily on textbooks, syllabi, or other artifacts to guide the course of study.

I believe that the four principles enunciated in this book are "brain-compatible," since they are consistent with the work on hemisphericity. However, I warn the reader once again that there is no empirical way to demonstrate that a specific teaching procedure is capable of activating a certain part of the brain *under normal teaching conditions* (short of hooking up each student to PET or fMRI equipment). Moreover, so little is known about the connection between brain activities and learning processes that it would be foolish to claim that a specific area of the brain is involved in carrying out a certain task. Nevertheless, the cautious view adopted in this book is that neuroscientifically-based procedures *can* enhance learning outcomes in a demonstrable way. The excursion into the neuroscientific domain on the part of some practitioners has, therefore, been anything but fanciful. It has forced us to look more closely at the conditions we create in a classroom, at the theoretical suppositions underlying instructional practices and teaching syllabi and, last but not least, at the actual techniques we use to carry out tasks.

The question of which *techniques* can be used to "activate the brain" in the classroom constitutes the subject matter of this final chapter. Actually, the techniques for doing so already exist. The principles discussed in this book suggest, essentially, how to select and adapt them. Specifically, they suggest that: (1) R-Mode techniques are required initially for imparting novel material; (2) L-Mode techniques must be used after this stage to consolidate learning; (3) specific techniques (R-Mode or L-Mode) to help students correct error patterns or to help them relearn something might be needed from time to time; (4) contextualization techniques are necessary to support L-Mode learning; and (5) techniques that bring out the relation between concepts and language forms are critical during both R-Mode and L-Mode stages.

Incidentally, the viability of developing such a framework was examined during the 2000-2001 academic year. The Italian teachers in two high schools in the city of Toronto were trained to organize their grade 10 classes according to the five criteria mentioned above. The teachers in two other schools were told to continue teaching as was their custom, using their textbooks in the usual fashion. The experimental teachers were instructed to use their textbooks as ancillary tools, rather than as basic formats imposing a sequential learning system on teacher and learner alike. A team of research assistants was made available to the experimental teachers to answer questions of course structure and technique appropriateness. At the end of the academic year the learners in all the four schools were tested with standard proficiency tests, taken primarily from the *ACTFL Proficiency Guidelines* (1986). The results were extremely interesting. Simply put, the two experimental classrooms fared significantly better on a battery of tests (from grammar competence to writing ability), with a 71% average overall, whereas the two control classrooms achieved a 59% average. Moreover, when compared in terms of the ACTFL Proficiency levels, the experimental classes reached (on average) the level 4 (= ability to use the language fluently and accurately in most situations), whereas the control classes reached the level 3 (= ability to speak the language with sufficient structural accuracy and vocabulary to participate effectively in most conversations). (There are 11 levels in the Guidelines—0, 0+, 1, 1+, 2, 2+, 3, 3+, 4, 4+, 5).

The *Human Information Processing Survey* (HIPS) (Taggart and Torrance 1984) was administered initially to assess the students' hemispheric style, so as to determine if this could be a factor in any outcome. The HIPS contains 40 multiple-choice items and is supposed to yield separate standard scores for the subjects' degree of left, right, and integrated hemispheric specialization. Although such categorizations result as somewhat artificial, and can even be misleading in my view, they nevertheless can be used to lend tentative support to any general learning outcomes that manifest themselves. By examining the individual standardized scores from the HIPS in relation to specific outcomes, the idea is simply to provide relevant information about the scores. In essence, it was found that hemispheric style had no effect on the outcomes, since a mixed number of RH, LH, and integrated individuals were found distributed throughout the experimental and control classes.

Whether or not these results can be claimed to have "scientific" validity is a moot point. The study was observational in nature—no more, no less. As indicated throughout this book, such studies have cumulatively lent support to the teaching framework being elaborated in this book.

Repertoire of Techniques

A *technique* is any procedure that can be used to help accomplish certain objectives or tasks in class. It can be an explanation of grammar, a type of exercise or activity, a test, etc. that has an identifiable R-Mode, L-Mode, or intermodal focus in its design. The main techniques can be categorized generically as follows (even though there is much overlap among the categories):

- *Structural Techniques.* The aim of these techniques is the development of some aspect of linguistic, communicative, or conceptual competence.
- *Visual Techniques.* These have the same objective of the structural techniques. However, they are based on visual imagery and thus entail R-Mode processes in tandem with L-Mode ones.
- *Ludic Techniques.* These are game-playing and problem-solving techniques that enhance linguistic, communicative, and conceptual learning.
- *Humor Techniques.* These are R-Mode techniques (jokes, cartoons, etc.) that promote conceptual fluency.
- *Role-Playing Techniques.* These are techniques that are applicable during intermodal stages of learning.

Needless to say, the SLT Dilemma cannot be solved by simply possessing a thorough knowledge of the repertoire of techniques that are available and a framework for amalgamating them. In no way does this guarantee that the brain will be activated in a profitable way. Significant learning outcomes can only be assessed over protracted periods of time. Moreover, the outcomes will never be homogeneous—some students will attain high levels proficiency earlier than others; others need more time to do so; others still may never reach more than the mid-levels of proficiency; and so on. There are simply too many factors involved in SLA, including the teacher-learner relation that is established, the needs of the students, their learning styles, etc. But this does not mean that pedagogy cannot make a difference in getting *most of the learners* to achieve high levels of proficiency. The various neuronal structures in the brain work in an integrated fashion, influencing each other reciprocally. During a flow stage, the entire neuronal-synaptic system is presumably operative, while during a focusing stage specific "inactive" areas of "modules" within that system are activated. Thus, the use of techniques in terms of the flow, focusing, contextualization, and conceptualization principles will, arguably, act on the entire brain, but will do so over a period of time.

Structural Techniques

The list of structural techniques is a long one. These include teacher explanations of grammar and vocabulary, classroom exercises such as fill-ins, completions, transformations (changing nouns from singular to plural, verbs from present to past, etc.), and activities such as writing and translation. Most have either an R-Mode or an L-Mode focus. Some are intermodal, such as the *dictation* technique and its variant the *cloze* technique (whereby a student must fill-in missing words on the basis of a given dictation or written text). Translation exercises are also highly intermodal. However, caution must be exercised in the use of entire translation texts because a high degree of conceptual competence must have developed in the learner, otherwise the activity will prove to be useless and, perhaps, even counterproductive. Contextualization makes it possible to provide R-Mode support to L-Mode tasks, making them highly intermodal. A teacher's explanation of grammar, for instance, can be rendered intermodal with the use of visual supports, a technique that has been used to great advantage by both the AVM and the Cognitive-Code Method.

The list of techniques that can be used to provide exercise, reinforcement, practice, and activity sessions for learners is a long and extensive one. The following is a sampling of commonly-used techniques for carrying out such sessions. (Note: Italian is used throughout as the SL):

Minimal Contrast Techniques (Main Focus: L-Mode)

Cosa sai? vs. *Cosa fai?*
("What do you know?" vs. "What are you doing?")
Thisbrings out the phonemic contrast between /s/ e /f/.

Quando parti? vs. *Quando partì*
("When are you leaving?" vs. "When did he/she leave?")
This brings out the morphological and semantic contrast between the present and past absolute tenses.

Comparison Techniques (Main Focus: L-Mode)

These involve explicit comparisons between structural features of the target and native languages:

ch in Italian = *ch* in certain English words: *chemistry*, *ache*, etc.

Recognition techniques (Main Focus: L-Mode)

These allow students to recognize structural features (phonological, grammatical, semantic, etc.):

Which are colors and which are flowers?

verde ("green")
margherita ("daisy")
azzurro ("blue")
rosa ("rose, pink")

Correction Techniques (Main Focus: L-Mode)

These allow students to reflect consciously on structural aspects of the SL.

Correct the following sentences (to show the correct use of the definite article in Italian):

Pizza è buona ("Pizza is good") - *La pizza è buona*.

Bambini italiani sono simpatici ("Italian kids are nice") - *I bambini italiani sono simpatici.*

Completions (Main Focus: Intermodal)

These activate recognition and expectancy processes in the learner:

Barista: ________, *signore. Desidera?* (" ________, sir. May I help you?") (answer: *Prego*)

Signore: *Prendo* _____ *caffè lungo.* ("I'll have _________ long coffee") (answer: *un*)

Contextualized Translation (Main Focus: Intermodal)

This type of translation task allows the learner to focus on meaning and function, rather than simply on form:

Ask a classmate the following questions in Italian:

What's your name? *(Come ti chiami?)*
How are you? *(Come stai?)*
Where are you from? *(Di dove sei?)*

Contextualized Sentence-Making Techniques (Main Focus: R-Mode or intermodal as the case may be)

These allow students to work on the relation between syntax and meaning:

Gianni/ristorante/Maria ("Johnny/restaurant/Mary") = *Gianni è in un ristorante con Maria* ("Johnny is in a restaurant with Mary")

Contextualized follow-up:

Dov'è Gianni? ("Where is Johnny?") - *È in un ristorante* ("He's in a restaurant.")

Con chi è? ("With whom is he?") - *È con Maria* ("He's with Mary")

Transformation Techniques (Main Focus: L-Mode)

These allow students simply to work with forms in patterned ways.

Ho fame ("I am hungry")
(tu, Marco, loro)

Anche tu hai fame ("You're also hungry")
Anche Marco ha fame ("Mark is also hungry")
Anche loro hanno fame ("They're also hungry")

Personalization Techniques (Main Focus: Intermodal)

These inject a personal element into structural practice:

Dove abiti? ("Where do you live?")

Ti piace abitare in un appartamento o in una casa? ("Do you prefer living in an apartment or a house?")

Informed Guessing Techniques (Main Focus: R-Mode)

These are techniques that involve induction of form and pattern:

Guess the female version of the following male names:

Model: *Pino*
Pina

Paolo
Michele

Problem-Solving Techniques (Main Focus: R-Mode)

Chi è la donna che ti chiede informazioni sul tuo passato? (la psicanalista)
("Who is the woman who asks you information on your past?" - the psychoanalyst")

Chi dipinge quadri? (l'artista)
("Who paints pictures?" - an artist)

Substitution Techniques (Main Focus: L-Mode)

These allow students to develop familiarity with such processes as anaphora and cataphora (chapter 4):

Replace noun phrases with appropriate object pronouns in answering the questions:

Hai mai studiato il francese? - Sì, l'ho studiato.
("Have you ever studied French? Yes, I have studied it.")

Sei mai andata in Francia? - Sì, ci sono andata due anni fa.
("Have you ever gone to France? - Yes I went there two years ago.")

Cloze Techniques (Main Focus: R-Mode)

These allow students to focus on the relation between structures, meaning, and discourse flow:

Ecco _________ *oroscopo.* ("Here's _________ horoscope.")
(answer: *il tuo* "your")

Domani avrai molto _________ *nelle scelte professionali..* ("Tomorrow you will have much _________ in your professional decisions.")

(answer: *successo* "success")

Multiple Choice Techniques (Main Focus: L-Mode or R-Mode as the case may be)

These constitute simple recognition exercises:

la macchina ("the car")

Si usa per andare in giro.
("We use it to get around.")

Comprehension Techniques (Main Focus: L-Mode)

These are useful follow-up L-Mode techniques that can be used after some novel learning task has been accomplished (performing a dialogue, reading a text, etc.):

Come si chiamano gli amici di Barbara?
("What are the names of Barbara's friends?")

Che cosa prende ciascuno di loro?
("What is each one having?")

Dove va ciascuno di loro?
("Where is each one going?")

Perché?
("Why?")

Content/Concept-Based Techniques (Main Focus: R-Mode)

These techniques impart conceptual competence:

• paraphrasing passages or texts;
• writing various kinds of texts on specific themes;
• making up realia (ads, comic strips, etc.);
• transforming a text written in one style into another (e.g. from a dialogue to a narrative);
• modifying or expanding texts in some creative way;
• comparing texts;
etc.

Visual Techniques

The first systematic use of visual techniques in SLT can be traced back to Comenius' textbook, the *Orbis sensualium pictus* of 1648. Visual techniques are those that either: (1) provide visual contexts to accompany the verbal input (as in cartoon strips with missing text), or else (2) provide illustrative support for some explanation, exercise, activity, etc. Audiovisual devices, such as videos, film strips, computer software of various kinds, can also be included in this category. The literature on the use of the latter is rather large and need not be discussed here. The interested reader can consult the relevant items in the bibliography at the back of this book. Suffice it to say, generally, that visual techniques not only support teaching, but also provide crucial R-Mode contextualization for learning. Here are just two examples of how visual images can be used practically for classroom tasks:

Identification Tasks

Per ogni figura, dare l'espressione che meglio esprime lo stato emozionale della persona.
("For each figure, give an expression that best fits the emotional state of the person")

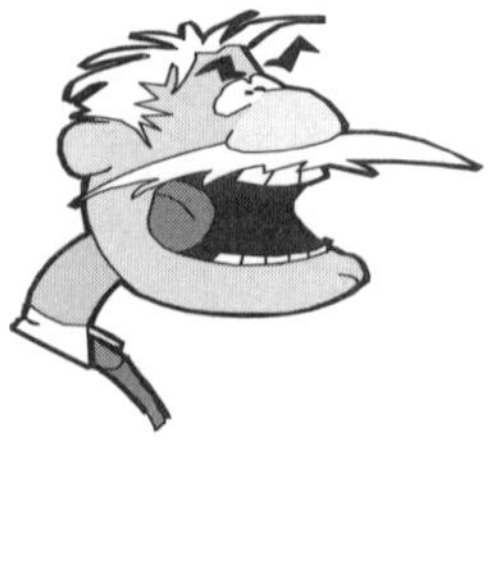

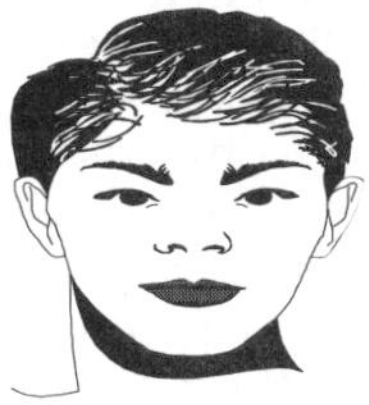

Grammar Tasks

Utilizzando il presente progressivo, descrivere quello che stanno facendo le seguenti persone.
("Using the present progressive, describe what the following people are doing")

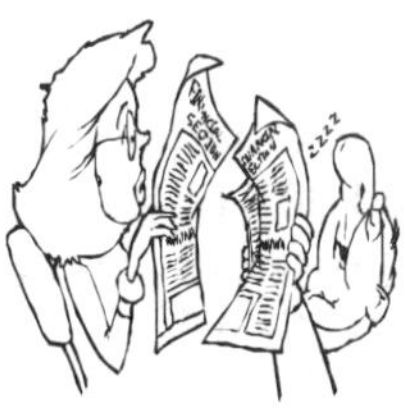

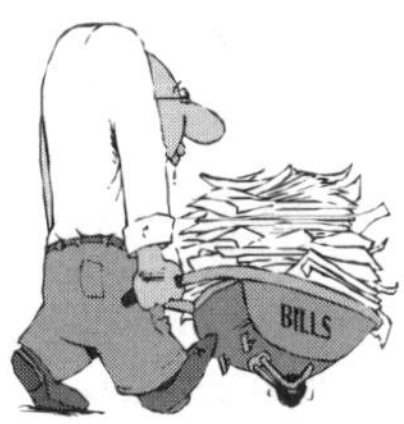

From the point of view of the conceptualization principle, it can be said that the more the visual imagery is illustrative of the conceptual domain being learned, the more likely will conceptual competence be fostered.

Ludic Techniques

Any game-playing or problem-solving technique can be classified as *ludic*. Since the 1960s, ludic materials such as crosswords, word searches, scrambled words, simulations, interactive games, board games, etc. have become intrinsic components of many SLT approaches, used especially for the review and reinforcement of grammar, vocabulary, and communication skills.

The experimental literature dealing with the learning-efficacy of such techniques is not extensive. Outside of a few scattered attempts to assess their validity and to develop a psychologically-appropriate typology for their instructional utilization, very little has been done in the way of giving the topic of ludic techniques a thorough empirical treatment. Two clear facts have nevertheless emerged from the sketchy literature and from anecdotal evidence. First, such techniques seem to be supportive of language acquisition processes. Second, for such techniques to be effective, they must be designed with specific instructional/learning objectives in mind. The general research in educational psychology, the corpus of case studies of learners, the everyday observations of school teachers, and the common perceptions of anyone in daily contact with learners point collectively to the efficacy of ludic techniques. They are easily inserted into the frameworks of most contemporary proficiency-oriented approaches because: (1) they foster language use; (2) they are rule-governed (i.e. they have a limited numbers of specific and clearly-defined rules); (3) they are goal-defined; (4) they have closure (i.e. there is a specific point at which a puzzle is solved or a game is finished); and (5) they are engaging, in that they constantly seem to challenge the participants.

Ludic techniques are thought by many practitioners to be "ancillary activities" that can be easily used in combination with other kinds of instructional techniques. Rarely has anyone ventured to design a syllabus, or teaching system, aimed at making the whole SLT process ludic in orientation. One of the few to have done so, as reported in his Ph.D. dissertation of 1992, is Mark Miller of the University of Delaware. Miller designed an entire syllabus and instructional system based on interactive game-playing. Using the usual experimental-statistical method of a controlled study, he found his game-playing design to be an effective means of imparting both linguistic and communicative competence to university language students, while at the same time allowing for the maintenance of a high level of interest and motivation in the course. While his project was designed only as a pilot study, it nonetheless gives substance to the claim that such techniques are effective *on their own*.

A distinction between *language teaching puzzles* (LTPs) and *language teaching games* (LTGs) should be maintained for pedagogical purposes, since the former are problem-solving texts that require the individual learner to come up with a solution, while the latter involve group-based problem-solving activities. Both kinds are useful for imparting conceptual competence because they require students to decipher the conceptual domains underlying the puzzle or game. Before selecting or preparing the specific LTPs or LTGs for classroom learning objectives, the teacher should always keep in mind that the preferences, learning styles, and backgrounds of the students must be taken into consideration. Most learners can handle LTPs that are cast in simplified form (e.g. elementary crosswords, word searches, etc.). But some have great difficulty in handling such LTPs as logic puzzles, rebuses, etc. Therefore, bearing in mind that LTPs and LTGs must be synchronized to the learners' abilities and level of competence, ludic techniques are useful for at least three reasons:

- Some LTPs promote L-Mode form-based language learning; others promote R-Mode conceptual learning. The former can be called *form-based* LTPs, the latter *concept-based* LTPs. LTGs promote R-Mode communication-based learning.

- Both LTPs and LTGs can be easily constructed and keyed to specific and general instructional objectives. Once the learning task has been determined, the teacher can select or construct the appropriate LTP or LTG to accomplish it.
- LTPs and LTGs should be used judiciously. They should never be used as "time-fillers." The learners should be made to understand that they are just as much a part of the course as are other kinds of exercises, drills, activities, etc. The teacher should also keep in mind that the over-use of LTPs and LTGs is not desirable. To maintain interest, the teacher should always diversify the types of LTPs and LTGs used together with other kinds of techniques.

Form-based LTPs direct the individual learner's attention to language form. They are among the most popular types of LTPs, and are found regularly in textbooks and ancillary textual materials. Scrambled letters, crosswords, word searches, tic-tac-toe puzzles, word mazes, cryptograms, and the like make up a truly rich and broad repertoire of LTPs that can be tailored to fit specific form-based learning tasks. Such LTPs are popular with both teachers and learners because they cast the reinforcement and control of spelling, grammar, and vocabulary into a challenging and recreational problem-solving format.

Form-based LTPs are highly versatile. The same LTP can be used for more than one objective. Take, as an example, the following word-search LTP, which has the Italian color adjectives *rosso, nero, bianco, verde,* and *giallo* hidden in it:

A	B	V	E	R	D	E	B	A	T	Y	U	I	O	N
A	D	R	T	Y	U	I	O	P	O	I	N	B	N	E
B	N	M	B	I	A	N	C	O	O	P	M	N	I	R
R	M	K	L	O	P	O	I	L	M	K	I	O	I	O
Y	G	I	A	L	L	O	M	O	I	U	R	N	L	M
B	N	I	O	L	A	N	B	N	M	O	O	I	R	O
G	E	R	Y	U	O	I	R	T	Y	M	S	N	M	K
A	Q	W	S	X	C	D	E	N	J	U	S	M	K	L
L	O	P	I	U	Y	T	M	P	O	L	O	N	T	Y

Figure 12. Search Puzzle

The words can be read from left-to-right, right-to-left, up-down, and down-up. Now, this puzzle can be used for a variety of review, control, and reinforcement objectives. Here are a few examples:

The students can be asked simply to locate the color adjectives in the puzzle, after having given them the words (= simple recognition task):

Trova le parole "bianco", "nero", "verde", "rosso" e "giallo" nel "puzzle"
("Find the words w.hite, black, green, red and yellow in the puzzle.")

The students can be asked to locate five color adjectives in the puzzle, without telling them which ones (= vocabulary review task):

Nel seguente "puzzle" ci sono cinque colori. Trovali.
("There are five colors in the puzzle. Find them.")

The students can be given incomplete sentences for each word and then asked to find the missing words in the puzzle (= cloze task):

Trova le parole mancanti nel puzzle.
("Find the missing words in the puzzle.")

L'erba è _______ ("The grass is _______")
Il sole è _______ ("The sun is _______")

The students can be given the feminine forms of the adjectives and then asked to locate their corresponding masculine forms in the puzzle (= morphological task):

Trova le forme maschili dei seguenti colori nel puzzle.
("Find the masculine forms of the following colors in the puzzle.")

rossa
verde

And so on.

The number and diversity of uses form-based LTPs can have is limited only by the imagination and specific requirements of the teacher. *Concept-based* LTPs, on the other hand, focus the learner's attention on meaning, and are thus especially useful for promoting conceptual fluency. Riddles, logical deductions, simple math puzzles, and the like fall into this category.

Consider, as an example, the following logical deduction puzzle:

> In a certain company, Bob, Janet, and Shirley hold the positions of director, engineer, and accountant, but not necessarily in that order. The accountant, who is an only child, earns the least. Shirley, who is married to Bob's brother, earns more than the engineer. What position does each person fill?

We are told that the accountant is an only child, but that Bob has a brother. So, clearly, we can eliminate Bob as the accountant. We are also told that the accountant earns the least of the three, but that Shirley earns more than the engineer does. From these two statements, we can establish two fairly obvious things about Shirley: (1) that she is not the accountant (who earns the least, while she earns more than someone else does); (2) that she is not the engineer (since she earns more than that person does). By the process of elimination, the *Accountant* is *Janet*. Since neither *Janet* nor *Shirley* is the Engineer; the *Engineer* must be *Bob*. This leaves *Shirley* as *Director*:

The important features about this type of LTP can be summarized in point form as follows:

- The learner must focus on the meaning-to-form relations that are inherent in the puzzle.
- The learner must make inferences in terms of the puzzle's language.
- As a consequence, concept-based LTPs tend to develop the learner's conceptual competence.

An LTG is useful during intermodal stages. No special commentary is required here because an LTG is akin to any role-laying technique, since it unfolds as a group-based, interactive task that focuses the learner's attention on language use and meaning negotiation. LTGs such as charades, *What's My Line?*, board games, card games, etc. create contexts in which the language is to be used in discourse-appropriate ways.

Humor Techniques

Techniques designed to evoke humor (jokes, cartoons, etc.) are useful for developing conceptual fluency. Again, it is not necessary here to delve into the many kinds of strategies, materials, and activities that can be used to evoke humorous reactions. Suffice it to say that they are in line with the contextualization and conceptualization principles. Take, as a simple example, the following Italian vignette:

Un signore entra in un bar ("A gentleman enters a bar").

Signore:	*Un bicchiere di vino, per favore!* ("A glass of wine, please!")
Barista:	*Rosso o bianco?* ("Red or white?")
Signore:	*Rosso!* ("Red!")
Barista:	*Dolce o secco?* ("Sweet or dry?")
Signore:	*Secco!* ("Dry!")
Barista:	*Locale o di marca?*

	("Local or brand-name?")
Signore:	*Locale!*
	("Local")
Barista:	*Di fiasco o di bottiglia?*
	("In a flask or a bottle?")
Signore:	*Non importa! Un caffè, per favore!*
	("Forget it! I'll have a coffee, please!"
Barista:	*Normale o macchiato?*
	("Normal or with a touch of milk?"
Signore:	*Normale!*
	("Normal!")
Barista:	*Ristretto o lungo?*
	(Strong or mild?
Signore:	*Ristretto!*
	("Strong")
Barista:	*Corretto o semplice?*
	("With a drop of alcohol or without?")

A questo punto, il signore scappa disperato! ("At this point, the gentleman runs away desperate!")

The humorous reaction that this dialogue will undoubtedly activate crucial R-Mode functions (chapter 2). This vignette can be complemented with typical follow-up exercises and content questions that involve the L-Mode and R-Mode in various ways:

Correggi ciascuna affermazione, seguendo il modello ("Correct each statement, following the model").

Model: *Un signore entra in una casa* ("house")
No, non entra in una casa, entra in un bar.

1. Desidera un bicchiere di vino bianco.
2. Desidera un bicchiere di vino dolce.
3. Desidera un bicchiere di vino di marca.
4. Desidera un caffè macchiato.
5. Desidera un caffè lungo.
6. Il signore rimane *(remains).*

Con un compagno/una compagna metti in scena una delle seguenti situazioni a piacere, imitando il dialogo ("With a partner, role-play one of the following scenes freely, imitating the dialogue").

Model: *cappuccino*

Signore/signorina:	*Un cappuccino, per favore.*
Barista:	*Caldo o freddo?*
Signore/signorina:	*Caldo.*
Barista:	*Amaro o dolce.*
Signore/signorina:	*Non importa! Non prendo niente.*

1. bicchiere di vino
2. caffè
3. tè
4. qualsiasi altra bevanda ("any other beverage")

Role-Playing Techniques

Role-playing techniques are pivotal in all Communicative Language Teaching approaches. Some of these are illustrated below. As mentioned throughout this book, they are designed to involve students in communicative exchanges during intermodal stages:

Pair Work

Chiedere ad un compagno come si chiama, come sta, ecc. ("Ask a partner what his/her name is, how he/she is, etc.")

Ordinare vari tipi di caffè in un bar.
("Order various types of coffee in a bar.")

Conversation-Making

In groups of three carry out conversations following the model:

Barista:	*Prego? Desiderano?* ("Yes? May I help you?")
Signore:	*Un cappuccino, per favore.* ("A cappuccino, please.")
Signora:	*Per me, invece. un'acqua minerale, grazie.* ("I'll have a mineral water instead, thanks.")
Barista:	*Prego. / Va bene.* ("Fine.").
Signora:	*Un momento, ho cambiato idea.* ("One moment please, I have changed my mind."

The techniques that involve the students in a creative fashion are particularly useful for intermodal learning (Di Pietro 1987). Here is a typical example:

Role A

Stai cercando di salire sull'autobus e inavvertitamente ti urti contro uno sconosciuto che ha dei pacchi ingombranti che cadono per terra. Che cosa gli dici? Ricorda che l'autobus sta per partire.

("You are trying to get on a bus and inadvertently you bump into a stranger with large packages which fall down. What would you say to him? Remember that the bus is about to leave.")

Role B

Hai appena comprato delle porcellane delicate ed uno sconosciuto ti urta facendo cadere tutti i pacchi a terra. Come reagirai?

("You have just bought some delicate pieces of porcelain and a stranger has bumped into you making the packages fall on the ground. How will you react?")

Organizational Issues

Issues of *selection* (what to teach) and *sequencing* (when to teach it) have always constituted the "sum and substance" of the traditional SLT methods and approaches. In a bimodal framework, these are not as critical as they are in other frameworks. Essentially, if an input or a task is new—i.e. if a structural or conceptual pattern to be learned or practiced is new and contrasts with the student's L1 or CS1—then the modal flow principle applies and the selection of items should be arranged to allow for a learning "flow" from the "R-Mode to the L-Mode," so to speak. During a focusing stage, on the other hand, either R-Mode or L-Mode techniques will be required depending on the pattern to be relearned, reinforced, corrected, or habitualized. An R-Mode technique is one that allows the learner an opportunity to experience the pattern in its totality without explanation or analysis. An L-Mode technique, on the other hand, is one that leads the learner to understand the reasons why the pattern is the way it is.

Needless to say, this puts more of the onus on the individual teacher's shoulders, rather than on some abstract methodical plan, textbook format, or syllabus design. Like a piano teacher, the language instructor will have to decide what and when to teach something, based on his/her observations of classroom behavior.

Selecting an Appropriate Technique

As mentioned in this and previous chapters, if a pattern or task is determined to be novel, then the modal flow principle applies. This involves the use of R-Mode techniques during the initial orientation period. The tradition established by the DM of using dialogues is, clearly, still a valid one in this regard. Humor techniques can also be used during R-Mode stages to promote conceptual fluency. However, the more the student knows about the L2 and the CS2, the less crucial is it to abide by the requirements of the modal flow principle, since enough L-Mode schemas are available to the learner to process the new input. The follow-up explanatory and practice stage is, of course, an L-Mode phase. Any structural, visual, or ludic technique can generally be used to meet the learning objectives of this stage. It depends on the nature of the course and the learning styles of the students. Allowing the students to apply the new pattern to creative role-playing constitutes the final intermodal phase. There is no evidence to suggest, incidentally, that role-playing techniques promote learning during orientation stages. They may, in fact, even be detrimental, leading to fossilized errors. Needless to say, reading and writing activities can also be used to promote intermodal learning.

Consider a case in point. Let us assume that "social contact" is the novel pattern in question. In elementary courses, a simple dialogue structured in a conceptually-appropriate fashion is, normally, a suitable R-Mode technique for starting the modal learning flow. The following one illustrates a culturally-appropriate way for young people to meet at a bar in Italy:

Maria: *Ciao, Claudia, che fai qui?*
("Hi, Claudia, what are you doing here?")

Claudia: *Prendo un caffè prima di andare a lavoro. E tu?*
("Having a coffee, before going to work. And you?")

Maria: *Anch'io.*
("Me too")

Claudia: *Che bella serata che abbiamo trascorso insieme sabato sera, no?*
("What a great night we spent together last Saturday, no?")

Maria: *Sì, mi sono veramente divertita.*
("Yeah, I really had fun.")

As a follow-up to the dialogue, the teacher can use various L-Mode structural techniques to allow the learner to grasp the new pattern. Here are some simple examples of techniques with which teachers of all methodological stripes are familiar:

True or false

Maria prende un caffè. ("Mary is having a coffee").

Claudia va a fare delle spese. ("Claudia is going to go shopping").

Le due amiche sono state ad una festa sabato sera. ("The two friends were at a party on Saturday night").

Completions

Claudia è in un _________. ("Claudia is in a _________")

Anche Maria è in un _________. ("Mary too I in a _________")

Claudia prende un _________. ("Claudia is having a _________")

Content Questions

Dove sono Claudia e Maria? ("Where are Claudia and Mary?")

Cosa prendono? ("What are they having"?)

Dove deve andare Claudia? ("Where does Claudia have to go?"

Paraphrases

Claudia e Maria sono in un _________. *Maria prende un* _________. *Anche Claudia prende un* _________. *ecc.*
("Claudia and Mary are in a _________. Mary is having a _________. Claudia too is having a __________. etc.).

Multiple Choices

Sabato sera Claudia......
a. *è andata ad una festa* b. *è andata al cinema* c. *è andata fuori città*
("Saturday night Claudia...... a. went to a party, b. went to the movies, c. went out of town")

Claudia sta per andare......
a. *al centro* b. *a lavoro* c. *a casa*
("Claudia is about to go...... a. downtown, b. to work, c. home")

Controlled Communication Activities

Saluta un amico/un'amica al bar. ("Greet a friend at a bar.")

Chiedigli/Chiedile perché si trova lì. ("Ask him/her why he/she is there").

For focusing and intermodal phases, there exists a vast repertoire of activities that can be used to promote communicative and conceptual competence. Here are a few of these activities:

Communication Tasks

Order the following beverages at a bar:

Model: *un caffè*
Vorrei un caffè, per favore. / Prendo un caffè, grazie.
("I would like a coffee, please / I'll have a coffee, thanks")

un caffè
un espresso
un cappuccino

Identification Tasks

Identify what the person is doing:

Model: *Un caffè, per favore*
(ordering a cup of coffee)

Ciao, Maria, come stai? ("Hi, Mary, how are you")
(Greeting someone)

Arrivederci, Paola. A domani. ("Good-bye Paula. See you tomorrow.")
(Taking leave of someone)

Pair Work

Greet the person sitting next to you:

Model: *Ciao, Debbie. Come stai?* ("Hi, Debbie. How are you?")
Bene, grazie. E tu? ("Fine, thanks. And You?")
Non c'è male. ("Not bad.")

Interactional Activities

Three students should carry out an encounter at a bar, extemporizing freely:

Model: Gianni / Carlo / Tina

Gianni: *Carlo, ti presento Tina.*
("Charles, let me introduce you to Tina.")

Carlo: *Piacere, Tina. Di dove sei?*
("A pleasure, Tina. Where are you from?")

Tina: *Sono di Milano. E tu?*
("I'm from Milan. And you?")

Carlo: *Io sono di qui.*
("I'm from here")

Functional Tasks

Create appropriate questions regarding the two persons in the dialogue:

Model: *Maria*
Dov'è Maria? / Che prende Maria?/ etc.
("Where is Mary? / What is she having?"/ etc.)

Personalization Activities

Indicate your personal preferences

Model: *il caffè espresso*
Sì, mi piace. / No, non mi piace.
("Yes, I like it. / No, I don't like it.")

il cappuccino
incontrare gli amici in un bar ("meeting friends in a bar")

Information-Giving Tasks

Ciascuno studente dovrà indicare il tipo di bevanda che prende di solito quando va al bar, con chi ci va, di che cosa parlano insieme, ecc.

("Each student should indicate what type of beverage he/she has usually in a bar, with whom he/she goes, what they usually talk about, etc.)

Information-Getting Tasks

Ask a partner what he/she usually has at a bar, with whom she/he likes to go, etc.

Grammatical Induction Tasks

Complete the following phone conversation with the verbs *potere, volere, dovere* ("to be able to, to want, to have to"):

Franco: *Maria, ________ venire stasera al bar Roma?*
("Mary, ________ to come this evening to the bar Roma?")

Maria: *No, Franco, non ________ venire.*
("No, Frank, I ________ come")

Descriptions

Describe what the following might wear to a bar.

un amico/un'amica sfarzoso (-a) ("a flamboyant friend")
un amico/un'amica antipatico (-a) ("a cranky friend")

Discussions

Answer the following questions.

Quante volte vaial bar alla settimana? ("How many times a week do you go to a bar?")

Perché? ("Why?")

Completions

Si va al bar per... ("One goes to a bar to ...")

Preferisco prendere un cappuccino, anziché un espresso ristretto, perché... ("I prefer a cappuccino, rather than a strong espresso, because...")

Conceptual Analysis

The use of *prendere* "to take" rather than *avere* "to have" as in English is a conceptual contrast:

Use *prendere* or *avere* as required by the situation:

Io _____ *tante lezioni* ("I have many classes")
Lui _____ *troppi caffè* ("He has too many coffees")
etc.

In sum, the selection and sequencing of techniques depends, as we have mentioned above and in other parts of this book, on the following:

During an R-Mode Stage

- R-Mode techniques should be used during initial orientation phases.
- The new input should thus be presented through simulations, dialogues, etc.
- The interactive participation of all students should be stressed.

During an L-Mode Phase

- The techniques should serve the teacher's objectives in bringing out the structural, communicative, and conceptual dimensions of the new input.
- The new material must be analyzed in a descriptive fashion.
- Repetition, imitation, reinforcement, etc. will be needed to allow the L-Mode to store the critical features of the new input.

During an Intermodal Phase

- The students will need to use the new information in creative ways.
- This is the phase during which ludic, humor, and game-playing techniques have the most utility.

- The teacher should step in only for modal focusing reasons (i.e. when he/she notices that some aspect needs reinforcement and special practice).

Integrating Linguistic, Communicative, and Conceptual Systems

Perhaps the most important aspect of Bimodality Theory is that a correlation between the linguistic, communicative, and conceptual systems must always be maintained. The following chart gives a few self-explanatory examples of how a certain conceptual theme, *time*, can guide the selection of the linguistic and communicative forms that *reflexivize* this theme in speech acts:

Table 7. Integrating Systems

Conceptual	Linguistic		Communicative
Metaforms	Vocabulary	Grammar	Speech Functions
time is a quantity	*l'una, le due,* *le tre,* etc. ("one o'clock, two o'clock, three o'clock") Expressions: *avere tempo* ("to have time") *perdere tempo* ("to waste time"), *acquistare tempo* ("to gain time")	The cardinal numbers Verbs such as: *avere* ("to have") *perdere* ("to lose")	Telling time *Che ore sono?* ("What time is it?") *Sono le tre* ("It's three o'clock")
time is a living entity	Expressions: *Il tempo vola* ("time flies") *Il tempo non perdona* ("time does not forgive")	Verbs such as: *volare* ("to fly") *perdonare* ("to forgive")	Discourse formulas, such as: *Il tempo non perdona nessuno!* ("Time forgives no one!")
time is a point	Expressions: *in futuro* ("in the future") *in passato* ("in the past"), *attualmente* ("at present")	Simple tense structures: the present tense the present perfect the future temporal adverbs	Connecting time events *Oggi = attualmente* ecc. ("today" = "at present")
time is an event/occurrence	*volta* ("time") *occasione* ("occasion, chance") *ogni tanto* ("every once in a while") *spesso* ("often")	Sequence of tenses	Referring to actions in sequence

Similar *reflexivization* charts can be easily envisioned for other domains of the CS2. In effect, these show how to integrate linguistic, communicative, and conceptual elements around a specific metaform. The role of testing in a bimodal framework should also be based on the notion of reflexivization. There is no need here to go into the theory of testing and the kinds of tests that can be used. The literature on this aspect of SLT is vast. Suffice it to say that testing should be introduced only as an evaluative component of what the student has acquired.

Concluding Remarks

The underlying theme of this book has been that SLT has gained considerably from its foray into the neuroscientific domain. But I also emphasize for the final time that this excursus has produced very little in the way of empirical research findings. Most neuroscientifically-designed methods of instruction have been based primarily on idiosyncratic extrapolations from the neuroscientific literature by highly dedicated teachers. So, I cannot help but agree with Obler (1983: 191) when she observes that, unless we are very careful, many unnecessary problems are bound to crystallize when extracting "too many implications from the work on hemisphericity."

Nevertheless, it is my fervent belief that neuroscientifically-based principles, such as the ones elaborated in this book, can put us all in a better position to tackle the SLT Dilemma in a systematic a way. Neuroscience has established that the brain's two hemispheres are designed anatomically to process information in a complementary fashion. Each hemisphere is specialized to handle a certain particular type of stimulus, but it does so in tandem with complementary or parallel processing patterns taking place in the other hemisphere and in other parts of the brain. The term "R-Mode" has been used in this book to refer to processes that have a primary locus in the RH, but which activate other areas of the brain in an interconnected fashion. Similarly, the term "L-Mode" has been used in reference to functions whose neural substrate is in the LH, but which receives information from other areas of the brain in a similarly interconnected fashion. The principles are derived from this interhemispheric model of brain functioning which asserts, basically, that new information is acquired in a "right-to-left" flow.

Needless to say, it would be just as foolish to claim that neuroscience provides the answers to solving the SLT Dilemma as it is to claim that psychology and linguistics do. We will probably never be able to solve the Dilemma with the theory-into-practice paradigm established by the reformers over a century ago, because of the complex biological, social, emotional, and conceptual nature of the overall learning task. But we can certainly try. Like good music teachers, experienced language teachers know all too well that each student is different, that each learning task presents its own kinds of problems and, thus, that *patience* is the operative word in all situations and contexts of learning.

My final thought is yet another caveat. No matter how scientific or theoretically sound a particular teaching proposal might appear to be, it is always susceptible to the vagaries of its human congener. The present one is no different. It is based on my own research and pedagogical experiences which, however, I firmly believe are reflective of the experiences of the "average classroom teacher."

GLOSSARY AND ABBREVIATIONS

A

Abstract concept	concept that cannot be demonstrated or observed directly
Afferent	receptive region of the brain
Alliteration	the repetition of the initial consonant sounds or features of words
ALM	Audiolingual Method
Anaphora	process of replacing previously-occurring words in a discourse text with other words or particles so that repetition can be attenuated or avoided
Anaphoric device	word or particle that refers back to a word uttered or written previously in a sentence or a discourse
Aphasia	partial or total loss of the ability to articulate words or comprehend spoken or written language, resulting from damage to the left hemisphere of the brain caused by injury or disease
Army Specialized Training Program	behaviorist language teaching method based on imitation and pattern practice, used to train army personnel during the Second World War
Association	process of connecting concepts with one another
Association cortex	any part of the cortex where information is analyzed, processed, or stored
Association-by-inference	associating concepts by a process of extension or perceived resemblance
Association-by-sense	associating concepts on the basis of perceived common features
Audiolingual Method	method devised in the 1940s on the behaviorist principle that the human learning system operated according to specific laws of habit formation

Audiovisual Method — European version of the ALM that made extensive use of visual props (filmstrips, photos, etc.)

AVM — Audiovisual Method

Axon — part of a nerve cell through which impulses travel away from the cell body

B

Basal ganglia — groups of neurons at the base of the cerebrum, helping to control well-learned movement sequences such as walking

Basic concept — concept having a typological function (also called **Prototypical concept**)

Behaviorism — school of psychology stressing the experimental study of observable behavior

Bilingualism — ability to use two languages with equal or nearly equal facility; method of education in which students who are not yet fluent in the language of the country where they live are taught in their native language

Bimodality — view of second language learning, espoused in this book, which claims that the functions associated with both hemispheres of the brain should be taken into account in second language teaching

Brain stem — lowest part of the brain, connecting the spinal cord with the cerebrum

Broca's Area — left hemispheric area responsible for speech, especially in its physical forms

C

CA — Contrastive Analysis

Cataphoric device — word or particle that anticipates a word in a sentence or discourse text

Cerebellum — part of the brain below the back of the cerebrum that regulates balance and movement and coordinates the muscles

Cerebral dominance — view that the left hemisphere of the brain is the dominant one for all the higher mental functions

Cerebral hemisphere	either the left or right side of the cerebrum
Cerebrum	largest and most complex portion of the brain that controls thought and learning
CF	conceptual fluency
CLT	Communicative Language Teaching
Cognitive style	the particular way in which information and knowledge are processed by an individual
Cognitive-Code Method	deductivist teaching method of the late 1960s and early 1970s stressing rule-learning and meaningful practice
Cognitivism	school of psychology stressing the study of mental processes independently of the physical behaviors they produce
Commisurotomy patients	patients who have had their corpus callosum separated to alleviate the pain associated with epileptic seizures (also called **Split-brain patients**)
Communication	capacity to participate with others in the exchange of meanings
Communicative competence	the ability to use language in specific situations
Communicative Language Teaching	movement stressing the teaching of the second language as a communicative tool, not as an abstract grammatical code to be learned independently of its communicative uses
Communicative syllabus	teaching syllabus organized according to the precepts of Communicative Language Teaching
Community Counseling	teaching method based on the idea that the students must be allowed to express their innermost feelings, and to choose what they want to learn in the target language
Complementarity theory	theory that the specific mental functions associated with each hemisphere of the brain work cooperatively in generating complex cognitive behaviors
Conceptual fluency	ability to use the conceptual system of a language in discourse
Conceptual ironic form	generalized ironical formula that defines a specific abstraction
Conceptual metaphor	generalized metaphorical formula that defines a specific abstraction
Conceptual metonym	generalized metonymic formula that defines a specific abstraction
Conceptual productivity	a measure of the frequency with which a specific concept occurs in a language

Concrete concept	concept that can be demonstrated or observed in a direct way
Concrete operations stage	stage from ages 7 to 12 when a child begins to deal with abstract concepts
Connotation	extension of the meanings of a concept
Context	the culture-specific information inhering in speech acts
Contextualization	term reflecting the widely-held view in second language teaching that meaningful contexts must always be provided for new input, practice routines, etc. in order for learning to be lasting
Contrastive Analysis	technique of comparing the structures and concepts of the SL and the NL
Corpus callosum	the largest bundle of nerve fibers connecting the left and right cerebral hemispheres
Cortex	deeply folded and ridged layer of neurons on the surface of the cerebrum
CP	conceptual productivity
CPH	Critical Period Hypothesis
Critical Period Hypothesis	hypothesis that language acquisition is completed by around the age of puberty
CS1	learner's native conceptual system
CS2	the conceptual system of the target culture

D

Deductivism	view that the grammar rules of the language should be taught first through explanation
Dendrite	structure at the receiving portion of a neuron
Denotation	concrete meaning of a concept
Diencephalon	posterior part of the forebrain that connects the mesencephalon with the cerebral hemispheres, encloses the third ventricle, and contains the thalamus and hypothalamus
Direct Method	language teaching method, developed in the late nineteenth century, based on the view that second language acquisition was equivalent to first language acquisition
DM	Direct Method
Dominance theory	view that the verbal left hemisphere is the dominant one in complex mental behaviors

E

EA Error Analysis

Efferent transmission region of the brain

Endbrain see **Telencephalon**

Error Analysis study of errors in the speech of second language learners

F

First language students' native language

fMRI Functional magnetic resonance imaging

Forebrain front part of the three primary divisions of the brain of a vertebrate embryo; part of the fully developed brain evolved from this, consisting of the diencephalon and the telencephalon

Formal operations stage stage from ages 12 to 15, when a child begins to reason logically and systematically

Frontal lobe region at the front and top of each cerebral hemisphere, important for reason, emotion, and judgment as well as voluntary movement

Functional magnetic resonance imaging new technology that enables neuroscientists to study healthy, living brains at work, producing images similar to X rays that show which parts of the brain are active while a person performs a particular mental or physical task; specifically. The fMRI images show the parts where high oxygen levels indicate increased activity, whereas PET (**Positron Emission Tomography**) images show the parts of the brain that are using the most glucose (a form of sugar).

G

Gambit verbal strategy for initiating or maintaining discourse flow

Ganglia group of nerve cells forming a nerve center, especially one located outside the brain or spinal cord

Generativism	school of linguistics based on the idea that grammar is a rule-governed system constituting an innate faculty of the brain
Glia	cells that form a supporting network for the neurons in the brain
Grammar-Translation Method	language teaching method stressing grammatical rule-learning and translation tasks
Ground	meaning of a metaphor
GT	Grammar-Translation
GTM	Grammar-Translation Method

H

Holophrase	one-word sentence uttered typically by infants around the age of 8-14 months
Hypothalamus	region in the upper part of the brain stem that controls body temperature, hunger, thirst, and the pituitary gland

I

Image schema	mental impression of locations, movements, shapes, etc.
Inductivism	view that grammar rules are best learned through induction
Input	samples of language (oral or written) to which a student is exposed in the classroom
Input Hypothesis	claim that the primary condition for second language acquisition is that the input to which students are exposed should consist of information that is a little bit beyond their acquired level of competence
Intake	the portion of **Input** that learners acquire
Interlanguage	type of speech manifested typically by second language learners, characterized by errors of certain types at different learning stages
Intermodal	functioning of the two main learning modes—the **L-Mode** and the **R-Mode**—in tandem
Irony	use of a word or statement that brings out meaning through contrast

Isomorphism	virtual synonymy between forms and concepts

L

L-Mode	left hemisphere learning mode
L1	learner's native language
L2	the target language
LAD	Language Acquisition Device
Language Acquisition Device	notion that language acquisition is governed by a mental faculty designed specifically for that purpose
Langue	theoretical knowledge of language
Lateral eye movement technique	experimental technique by which the movement of the eyes are videotaped. This is used to provide information on which hemisphere is involved in processing a specific kind of stimulus, given that in most people the activation of left-hemispheric functions causes the eyes to orient slightly to the right, while leftward orientation ensues from the activation of right-hemispheric functions.
Lateralization	natural process by which language is localized, in general, to the left hemisphere of the brain during childhood
Lesion	any damage to a brain area
LH	left hemisphere
Limbic system	primitive part of the brain near the brain stem thought to control emotions, behavior, smell, etc.
Linguistic competence	knowledge of language as a system
Linguistic performance	knowledge of how to use a language
Localization theory	theory that a specific mental function is localized in one specific area of the brain
LTG	language teaching game
LTP	language teaching puzzle

M

Medulla oblongata	lowest part of the brain stem, at the top end of the spinal cord, that regulates heartbeat, breathing, and other automatic functions

Mesencephalon portion of the vertebrate brain that develops from the middle section of the embryonic brain (also called the **Midbrain**)

Meta-metaform abstract concept that emerges from the linkage of different metaforms to each other

Metaform abstract concept that results from the linkage of an abstract target domain with a concrete source domain

Metaphor figure of speech containing an implied comparison, in which a word or phrase ordinarily and primarily used of one thing is applied to another

Metasymbol symbol derived from the constant association of metaforms to each other

Method language teaching system drafted according to a specific psychological theory of learning

Metonymy use of an entity to refer to another that is related to it

Midbrain see **Mesencephalon**

Modal flow view that flow" of learning should go from R-Mode learning to L-Mode focusing

Modal focusing view that at certain points in the learning process students will need to focus on one mode or the other (R-Mode or L-Mode)

Morpheme minimal meaning-bearing form in a language

Motor cortex part of both frontal lobes of the brain that controls voluntary muscle movements

Myelin fatty substance that surrounds and protects certain nerve fibers

N

NA Natural Approach

Natural Approach teaching method that stresses R-Mode learning techniques

Natural order view that there is a sequence of stages through which second language acquisition must pass

Negative transfer transfer of a native language feature to the learning of the target that interferes with the learning process

Neurolinguistic Method teaching method based on neurolinguistic principles, insights, and research findings

Neurolinguistics	branch of neuroscience aiming to investigate how language is organized and processed by the brain
Neuron	fundamental cellular unit of the nervous system
Neuroscience	discipline studying the brain
Neurotransmitters	chemicals that transmit nerve impulses between neurons
NL	native language
NLA	native language acquisition
NLM	Neurolinguistic Method
Notional-Functional Syllabus	language teaching syllabus devised in the early 1970s utilizing notional concepts

O

Occipital lobe	posterior lobe of each cerebral hemisphere, having the shape of a three-sided pyramid and containing the visual center of the brain
Occipital lobe	region at the back of each cerebral hemisphere that contains the centers of vision
Oral/Situational Method	method developed in the 1930s stressing the situational practice of new notions and structures

P

Parallel Distributed Processing	computer model of brain functioning aiming to show how systems in the brain purportedly interact with each other
Parietal lobe	middle lobe of each cerebral hemisphere between the frontal and occipital lobes; contains important sensory centers
Parole	knowledge of how to use a language
PDP	Parallel Distributed Processing
Personalization	view that a congenial classroom atmosphere should be sustained throughout a course, and that the learner's personal opinions, background experiences, etc. be invoked in the exercise and activity components of the course
PET	Positron Emission Tomography

Phoneme	minimal unit of sound in a language that allows its users to differentiate word meanings
PI	productivity index
Plasticity	brain's ability to renew destroyed or injured tissue, and to adapt to all kinds of input easily during childhood
Pons	part of the brain stem that joins the hemispheres of the cerebellum and connects the cerebrum with the cerebellum
Positive transfer	transfer of a native language feature to the learning of the second language that enhances the learning process
Positron Emission Tomography	new technology that enables neuroscientists to study healthy, living brains at work, producing images similar to X rays that show which parts of the brain are active while a person performs a particular mental or physical task; specifically, PET shows the parts of the brain that are using the most glucose (a form of sugar), whereas fMRI (**Functional magnetic resonance imaging**) shows the parts where high oxygen levels indicate increased activity
Pre-operational stage	stage from ages 2 to 7 when a child is preoccupied with verbal skills
Productivity Index	the number of source domains used to deliver a concept
Proficiency	ability to use the second language in an autonomous manner
Proficiency movement	second language teaching movement stressing an integration of linguistic and communicative syllabi
Prototypical concept	see **Basic concept**

R

R-Mode	right hemisphere learning mode
Reading Method	method popular in the 1920s and 1930s which stressed the attainment of reading skills
Reform Movement	educational movement stressing the use of inductive learning in the language classroom
Relative Productivity Index	A comparative measure of the Productivity Indexes for a specific concept in two language. It is the quotient that emerges when the lower PI is divided into the higher one.

Reticular formation	network of nerve cells deep within the brain stem that plays a major role in maintaining sleep or wakefulness
RH	right hemisphere
RPI	relative productivity index

S

Scenario Approach	teaching approach based on allowing students to contrive and perform their own dialogues
SDI	source domain productivity
Séance	in **Suggestopedia**, period during which students relax and sit comfortably in reclining chairs listening to background music while new language material is introduced
Second language	any language learned after the first, or native, language
Second language acquisition	unconscious learning of the second language
Second language teaching	teaching of second languages in a classroom environment
Sensorimotor stage	stage from birth to age 2 marked by a child's gaining motor control and learning about physical objects
Sensory cortex	any part of the brain that receives messages from the sense organs or messages of touch and temperature from throughout the body
Silent Way	method based on the idea that teaching must be subordinated to learning
SL	second language
SLA	second language acquisition
SLI	specific language impairment
SLT	second language teaching
Somatosensory cortex	area of the sensory cortex in the parietal lobes that receives messages of touch, temperature, and certain other bodily sensations
Source domain	set of vehicles (concrete forms) used to deliver the meaning of an abstract concept
Source Domain Productivity	a comparative measure of the vehicles utilized within source domains: e.g. the *seeing* source domain above is highly productive in English and Italian for the delivery of *thinking*; however, the *moving things* one is rather limited in both languages, since very few vehicles in the

	domain are selected to deliver the concept. Within each source domain, there are subdomains that provide the concept-user with an array of specific vehicles that can be utilized to provide subtle detail to some concept. The higher the SDP, the more likely the utilization of that source domain.
Specific Language Impairment	genetically-based inability to learn and use morphemes and other grammatical structures
Speech act	speech used to accomplish some objective or action
Split-brain patients	see **Commisurotomy patients**
Structural syllabus	language teaching syllabus in which grammatical structures are arranged in order of increasing complexity
Structuralism	school of linguistics aiming to study language as a system of structures
Subliminal learning	unconscious learning
Subordinate concept	concept needed for specialized purposes
Suggestopedia	NLM based on subliminal learning principles
Superordinate concept	concept with a highly general referential function
Supplementary speech area	area of the left hemisphere involved in some speech functions
Syllabus	compendium of items to be learned in a language course
Synapse	junction point of two neurons, across which a nerve impulse passes

T

Tag question	form added to the end of a sentence that is designed to seek consent, agreement, etc.
Target domain	what a metaform is about
Target language	language that a learner is attempting to learn
Technique	specific instructional activity or routine
Telegraphic stage	stage of language acquisition characterized by the making of brief phrases resembling telegraphic messages
Telencephalon	anterior portion of the forebrain, constituting the cerebral hemispheres and related parts (also called **Endbrain**)

Temporal lobe region at the lower side of each cerebral hemisphere, containing centers of hearing and memory

Thalamus structure at the top of the brain stem that serves as a relay center for sensory information

Threshold Level communicative teaching syllabus devised in the early 1970s by scholars commissioned to do so by the Council of Europe

Topic the subject of a metaphor

Total Physical Response NLM based on the idea that the R-Mode should dominate all phases of acquisition

TPR Total Physical Response

Transfer theory view that second language acquisition unfolds as a process characterized by the transfer of native language habits, forms, categories, etc. to the second language

U

UG Universal Grammar

Unimodality method that focuses on one of the two modes of learning (L-Mode or R-Mode)

Universal Grammar set of principles that define language which are purported to be present in the brain at birth

V

Vehicle part of the metaphor that is associated with the topic

W

Wernicke's area area of the left hemisphere responsible for language content and meaning

Williams syndrome genetic disorder that affects both body and brain, giving those who have it a strange and incongruous jumble of deficits and strengths. They have diminished cognitive capacities and heart problems, and age prematurely; yet they have outgoing personalities and a flair for language, showing an immense knowledge of language. However, they show problems in the selection of the appropriate words.

WORKS CITED AND GENERAL BIBLIOGRAPHY

The following bibliography includes both the works cited in the text and, more generally, the works that have constituted the research and theory background to my treatment of the various topics. It can thus be consulted as a general reading list.

A

Adams, J. L. (1986). *Conceptual Blockbusting*. Reading, Mass.: Addison-Wesley.

Agard, F. and Di Pietro, R. J. (1965a). *The Sounds of English and Italian.* Chicago: University of Chicago Press.

Agard, F. and Di Pietro, R. J. (1965b). *The Grammatical Structures of English and Italian.* Chicago: University of Chicago Press.

Albert, M. and Obler, L. K. (1978). *The Bilingual Brain.* New York: Academic.

Allen, J. B. P. (1983). A Three-level Curriculum Model for Second Language Education. *Canadian Modern Language Review* 4: 23-43.

Allen, J. B. P. (1988). The Development of Instructional Models in Second Language Education. *Annual Review of Applied Linguistics* 9: 179-192.

Allport, G. W. (1965). *Pattern and Growth in Personality.* New York: Holt.

Allwood, J. and Gärdenfors, P. (1998) (eds.). *Cognitive Semantics: Meaning and Cognition.* Amsterdam: John Benjamins.

American Council on the Teaching of Foreign Languages (1986). *ACTFL Proficiency Guidelines.* Hastings-on-Hudson, NY: ACTFL.

Anderson, J. A. (1983). *The Architecture of Cognition.* Cambridge, Mass.: Harvard University Press.

Andrews, E. (1990). *Markedness Theory.* Durham: Duke University Press.

Anthony, E. M. (1963). Approach, Method and Technique. *English Language Teaching* 17: 63-67.

Antinucci, F. (1971). Modelli dell'apprendimento linguistico. *Neurologia, Neuropsicologia e Psichiatria* 3: 157-192.

Anttila, R. (1977). *Analogy.* The Hague: Mouton.

Appelbaum, D. (1990). *Voice.* Albany: State University of New York Press.

Arbib, M. A. (1982). From Artificial Intelligence to Neurolinguistics. In M. A. Arbib, D. Caplan and E. Marshall (eds.), *Neural Models of Language Processes*, 77-94. New York: Academic.

Archibald, J. (200) (ed.). *Second Language Acquisition and Linguistic Theory.* London: Blackwell.

Ardila, A. (1984). Right Hemisphere Participation in Language. In: A. Ardila and F. Ostrosky-Solis (eds.), *The Right Hemisphere: Neurology and Neuropsychology*, 99-107. New York: Gordon and Breach.

Argyle, M. (1988). *Bodily Communication.* New York: Methuen.

Aristotle. (1952a). *Rhetoric.* In *The Works of Aristotle*, Vol. 11, W. D. Ross (ed.). Oxford: Clarendon Press.

Aristotle. (1952b). *Poetics.* In *The Works of Aristotle*, Vol. 11, W. D. Ross (ed.). Oxford: Clarendon Press.

Armstrong, T. (1994). *Multiple Intelligences in the Classroom.* Alexandria, Va.: Association for Supervision and Curriculum Development.

Arndt, H. and Pesch, H. W. (1984). Nonverbal Communication and Visual Teaching Aids: A Perceptual Approach. *Modern Language Journal* 68: 28-36.

Arnheim, R. (1969). *Visual Thinking*. Berkeley: University of California Press.

Arnò, L. (1994). *La bimodalità nell'apprendimento di una lingua straniera*. Dissertation, Università Cattolica del Sacro Cuore di Milano.

Arries, J. F. (1994). Constructing Culture Study Units: A Blueprint and Practical Tools. *Foreign Language Annals* 27: 523-534.

Asch, S. (1955). On the Uses of Metaphor in the Description of Persons. In: H. Werner (ed.), *On Expressive Language*, 29-39. Worcester: Clark University Press.

Asch, S. (1958). The Metaphor: A Psychological inquiry. In: R. Tagiuri and L. Petrullo (eds.), *Person Perception and Interpersonal Behavior*, 28-42. Stanford: Stanford University Press.

Asher, J. J. (1965). The Strategy of the Total Physical Response: An Application to Learning Russian. *International Review of Applied Linguistics* 3: 292-299.

Asher, J. J. (1969). The Optimal Age to Learn a Foreign Language. *Modern Language Journal* 53: 334-341.

Asher, J. J. (1972). Children's First Language as a Model for Second Language Learning. *Modern Language Journal* 56: 133-139.

Asher, J. J. (1977). *Learning Another Language Through Actions: The Complete Teacher's Guidebook.* Los Gatos: Sky Oaks.

Asher, J. J. (1981). The Total Physical Response: Theory and Practice. In: H. Wintz, (ed.), *Native Language and Foreign Language Acquisition*, 324-331. New York: New York Academy of Sciences.

Asher, J. J. (1988). *Brainswitching: A Skill for the 21st Century.* Los Gatos: Sky Oaks Productions.

Asher, J. J. (1988). *Brainswitching: A Skill for the 21st Century.* Los Gatos: Sky Oaks.

Asher, J. J., Kuudo, J. A. and De la Torre, R. (1974). Learning a Second Language through Commands: The Second Field Test. *Modern Language Journal* 58: 24-32.

Austin, J. L. (1962). *How to Do Things with Words.* Cambridge, Mass.: Harvard University Press.

Ausubel, D. A. (1965). Adult vs. Children in Second Language Learning: Psychological Considerations. *Modern Language Journal* 48: 420-424.

Ausubel, D. A. (1967). *Educational Psychology: A Cognitive View.* New York: Holt, Rinehart and Winston.

B

Bailey, K. (1998). *Learning about Language Assessment: Dilemmas, Decisions, and Directions.* Boston: Heinle & Heinle.

Bailey, K. and Nuna, D. (1996). *Voices from the Language Classroom: Qualitative Research in Second Language Education.* Cambridge: Cambriidge University Press.

Bailey, K. M. (1985). Classroom-Centered Teaching and Learning. In: M. Celce-Murcia (ed.), *Beyond Basics*, 109-123. Rowley, Mass.: Newbury House.

Balboni, P. (1991). *Tecniche didattiche e processi di apprendimento linguistico.* Padova: Liviana Editrice.

Balboni, P. (1994). *Didattica dell'italiano a stranieri.* Roma: Bonacci.

Bancroft, J. (1972). Foreign Language Teaching in Bulgaria. *Canadian Modern Language Review* 28: 9-13.

Bancroft, J. (1978). The Lozanov Method and Its American Applications. *Modern Language Journal* 62: 167-175.

Bancroft, J. (1995). *The Two-Sided Mind: Teaching and Suggestopedia*. Washington: Eric Clearing House.

Barasch, R. M. and Vaughan, J. C. (1994) (eds.). *Beyond the Monitor Model. Comments on Current Theory and Practice in Second Language Acquisition*. Boston: Heinle and Heinle.

Barcelona, A. (1999) (ed.). *Metaphor and Metonymy at the Crossroads: A Cognitive Perspective*. Berlin: Mouton de Gruyter.

Bardovi-Harlig, K. and Hartford, B. (1997). *Beyond Methods: Components of Second Language Teachers Education*. New York: McGraw-Hill.

Bashear, L. (1988). *Metalinguistic Awareness in Classroom FL Learning: Implications for Treating Grammar in an Interactive Method*. Dissertation, University of Delaware.

Battistella, E. L. (1990). *Markedness: The Evaluative Superstructure of Language*. Albany: State University of New York Press.

Beeman, M. (1993). Semantic Processing in the Right Hemisphere May Contribute to Drawing Inferences from Discourse. *Brain and Language* 44: 80-120.

Behrens, S. J. (1989). Characterizing Sentence Intonation in a Right Hemisphere Damaged Population. *Brain and Language* 37: 181-200.

Benedict, H. (1979). Early Lexical Development: Comprehension and Production. *Journal of Child Language* 6: 183-200.

Benton, A. L. (1964). Contributions to Aphasia before Broca. *Cortex* 3: 314-327.

Berk, L. E. (1994). Vygotsky's Theory: The Importance of Make-Believe Play. *Young Children* 50: 30-39.

Berko, J. (1958). The Child's Learning of English Morphology. *Word* 14: 150-177.

Berlin, B. and Kay, P. (1969). *Basic Color Terms*. Berkeley: University of California Press.

Bialystock, E. (1990). *Communication Strategies: A Psychological Analysis of Second Language Use*. London: Blackwell.

Bialystock, E. (1991) (ed.). *Language Processing in Bilingual Children*. Cambridge: Cambridge University Press.

Bialystock, E. (2001). *Bilingualism in Development: Language, Literacy, and Cognition*. Cambridge: Cambridge University Press.

Bialystock, E. and Hakuta, K. (1994). *In Other Words: The Science and Psychology of Second-Language Acquisition*. New York: Basic.

Birdsong, D. (1999) (ed.), *Second Language Acquisition and the Critical Period Hypothesis*. Mahwah, N. J.: Lawrence Erlbaum.

Birdwhistell, R. (1970). *Kinesics and Context: Essays on Body Motion Communication*. Harmondsworth: Penguin.

Black, M. (1962). *Models and Metaphors*. Ithaca: Cornell University Press.

Blair, R. W. (1982) (ed.). *Innovative Approaches to Language Teaching*. Rowley Mass.: Newbury House Publishers.

Blasko, D. and Connine, C. (1993). Effects of Familiarity and Aptness on Metaphor Processing. *Journal of Experimental Psychology: Learning, Memory, and Cognition* 19: 295-308.

Bloom, A. H. (1981). *The Linguistic Shaping of Thought: A Study in the Impact of Language on Thinking in China and the West*. Hillsdale, N. J.: Lawrence Erlbaum Associates.

Bloomfield, L. (1933). *Language*. New York: Holt.

Bloomfield, L. (1942). *Outline Guide for the Practical Study of Foreign Languages*. Baltimore: Linguistic Society of America.

Bloor, T. (1986). What Do Language Students Know about Grammar? *British Journal of Language Teaching* 24: 157-160.

Bogen, J. E. (1975). Some Educational Aspects of Hemispheric Specialization. *UCLA Educator* 12: 24-32.

Bogen, J. E., DeZure, R., Tenhouten, W. D. and Marsh, J. F. (1972). The Other Side of the Brain: The A/P Ratio. *Bulletin of the Los Angeles Neurological Societies* 37: 49-61.

Booth, W. (1979). Metaphor as Rhetoric: The Problem of Evaluation. In: S. Sacks (ed.), *On Metaphor*, 47-70. Chicago: University of Chicago Press.

Boswood, T. (1997). *New Ways of Using Computers in Language teaching*. Alexandria, Va.: Teachers of English to Speakers of Other Languages.

Bottini, G. *et al.* (1994). The Role of the Right Hemisphere in the Interpretation of Figurative Aspects of Language: A Positron Emission Tomography Activation Study. *Brain* 117: 1241-1253.

Boysson-Bardies, B. de and Vihman, M. M. (1991). Adaptation to Language: Evidence from Babbling and First Words in Four Languages. *Language* 67: 297-319.

Braine, M. (1963). The Ontogeny of English Phrase Structure: The First Phase. *Language* 39: 1-13.

Braine, M. (1971). The Acquisition of Language in Infant and Child. In: C. E. Reed (ed.), *The Learning of Language*, 34-56. New York: Appleton-Century-Crofts.

Bressan, D. (1970). Crossword Puzzles in Modern Language Teaching. *Audio-Visual Language Journal* 8: 93-95.

Bressan, D. (1987). Enigmatic Devices in English-Italian Translation. *Multilingua* 6: 69-75.

Brière, E. J. (1968). *A Psycholinguistic Study of Phonological Interference*. The Hague: Mouton.

Brinton, D. M. and Master, P. (1997). *New Ways in Content-Based Instruction*. Alexandria, Va.: Teachers of English to Speakers of Other Languages.

Britton, B. K. and Pellegrini, A. D. (1990) (eds.). *Narrative Thought and Narrative Language*. Hillsdale, N. J.: Lawrence Erlbaum Associates.

Britton, J. (1970). *Language and Learning*. Harmondsworth: Penguin.

Broca, P. (1861). Remarques sur le siège de la faculté du langage articulé suivies d'une observation d'aphémie. *Bulletin de la Société d'Anatomie* 36: 320-357.

Brooks, N. (1960). *Language and Language Learning: Theory and Practice*. New York: Harcourt, Brace.

Broselow, E. (1988). Second Language Acquisition. In: F. J. Newmeyer (ed.), *Language: Psychological and Biological Aspects*, 194-209. Cambridge: Cambridge University Press.

Broselow, E. (1988). Second Language Acquisition. In: F. J. Newmeyer (ed.), *Language: Psychological and Biological Aspects*, pp. 194-209. Cambridge: Cambridge University Press.

Brown, C. M. and Hagoort, P. (1999) (eds.). *The Neurocognition of Language*. New York: Oxford University Press.

Brown, H. D. (1994). *Principles of Language Learning and Teaching*. Englewood Cliffs, N. J.: Prentice-Hall.

Brown, H. D. (2001). *Teaching by Principles: An Interactive Approach to Language Pedagogy*. White Plains: Addison-Wesley.

Brown, H. D. and Gonzo, S. (1995) (eds.). *Readings on Second Language Acquisition*. Englewood Cliffs, NJ: Prentice Hall Regents.

Brown, R. (1958a). *Words and Things: An Introduction to Language*. New York: The Free Press.

Brown, R. (1958b). How Shall a Thing Be Called? *Psychological Review* 65: 14-21.

Brown, R. (1970). *Psycholinguistics*. New York: Free Press.

Brown, R. (1973.). *A First Language*. Cambridge, Mass.: Harvard University Press.

Brown, R. (1976). Reference: In Memorial Tribute to Eric Lenneberg. *Cognition* 4: 125-153.

Brown, R. (1986). *Social Psychology*. New York: Free Press.

Brown, R., Leiter, R. A., and Hildum, D. C. (1957). Metaphors from Music Criticism. *Journal of Abnormal and Social Psychology* 54: 347-352.

Brownell, H. H. (1988). Appreciation of Metaphoric and Connotative Word Meaning by Brain-Damaged Patients. In: C. Chiarello (ed.), *Right Hemisphere Contributions to Lexical Semantics*, 19-32. New York: Springer.

Brownell, H. H., Potter, H. H., and Michelow, D. (1984). Sensitivity to Lexical Denotation and Connotation in Brain-Damaged Patients: A Double Dissociation? *Brain and Language* 22: 253-265.

Bruner, J. (1983). *Child Talk*. New York: W. W. Norton.

Bruner, J. (1986). *Actual Minds, Possible Worlds*. Cambridge, Mass.: Harvard University Press.

Bruner, J. (1990). *Acts of Meaning*. Cambridge, Mass.: Harvard University Press.

Bühler, K. (1934). *Sprachtheorie: Die Darstellungsfunktion der Sprache*. Jena: Fischer.

Burt, M. K and Kiparsky, C. (1972). *The Gooficon: A Repair Manual for English*. Rowley, Mass.: Newbury House.

Byram, M. (1989). *Cultural Studies in Foreign Language Education*. Philadelphia: Multilingual Matters, Ltd.

Byrnes, H. (1998) (ed.). *Learning Foreign and Second Languages: Perspectives in Research and Scholarship*. New York: Modern Language Association.

C

Calvin, W. H. and Ojemann, G. A. (1994). *Conversations with Neil's Brain: The Neural Nature of Thought and Language*. New York: Addison-Wesley.

Cameron, L. and Low, G. (1999). *Researching and Applying Metaphor*. Cambridge: Cambridge University Press.

Canale, M. (1984). On Some Theoretical Frameworks for Language Proficiency. In: C. Rivera (ed.), *Language Proficiency and Academic Achievement*, 28-40. Clevedon: Multilingual Matters.

Canale, M. and Swain, M. (1979). *Communicative Approaches to Second Language Teaching and Testing*. Toronto: Ontario Ministry of Education.

Capelle, J. and Capelle, G. (1969). *La France en direct*. Waltheim, Mass.: Ginn.

Caplan, D. (1987). *Neurolinguistics and Linguistic Aphasiology*. Cambridge: Cambridge University Press.

Caplan, D. (1992). *Language: Structure, Processing and Disorders*. Cambridge, Mass.: MIT Press.

Caré, J. M. and Debyser, F. (1978). *Jeu, langage et creativité*. Paris: Hachette.

Carroll, J. B. (1971). Current Issues in Psycholinguistics and Second Language Teaching. *TESOL Quarterly* 5: 273-280.

Carroll, J. B. (1981). Conscious and Automatic Processes in Language Learning. *Canadian Modern Language Review* 37: 462-474.

Carroll, S. and Meisel, J. M. (1990). Universals and Second Language Acquisition. *Studies in Second Language Acquisition* 12: 201-208.

Carroll, S. E. (2001). *Input and Evidence: The Raw Material of Second Language Acquisition*. Amsterdam: John Benjamins.

Carter, R. (1999). *Vocabulary: Applied Linguistic Perspectives*. London: Routledge.

Celce-Murcia, M. (1991). Grammar Pedagogy in Second and Foreign Language Teaching. *TESOL Quarterly* 25: 459-480.

Celce-Murcia, M. (1991). Grammar Pedagogy in Second and Foreign Language Teaching. *TESOL Quarterly* 25: 459-480.

Changeaux, J. P. and Dehaene, S. (1989). Neural Models of Cognitive Functions. *Cognition* 33: 63-109.

Chastain, K. (1971). *The Development of Modern Language Skills: Theory to Practice*. Philadelphia: Center for Curriculum Development.

Chastain, K. (1975). Affective and Ability Factors in Second Language Acquisition. *Language Learning* 24: 153-161.

Cherwitz, R. and Hikins, J. (1986). *Communication and Knowledge: An Investigation in Rhetorical Epistemology*. Columbia: University of South Carolina Press.

Chesterman, A. (1998). *Contrastive Functional Analysis*. Amsterdam: John Benjamins.

Chiarello, C. (1988a). Semantic Priming in the Intact Brain: Separate Roles for the Right and Left Hemispheres? In: C. Chiarello (ed.), *Right Hemisphere Contributions to Lexical Semantics*, 59-69. Berlin: Springer.

Chiarello, C. (1988b) (ed.). *Right Hemisphere Contributions to Lexical Semantics*. Berlin: Springer.

Chiarello, C., Richards, L. and Pollack, A. (1992). Semantic Additivity and Semantic Inhibition: Dissociative Processes in the Cerebral Hemispheres? *Brain and Language* 42: 52-76.

Chomsky, N. (1957). *Syntactic Structures.* The Hague: Mouton.

Chomsky, N. (1964). Degrees of Grammaticalness. In: J. A. Fodor and J. J. Katz (eds.), *The Structure of Language*, 384-389. Englewood Cliffs, N. J.: Prentice-Hall.

Chomsky, N. (1965). *Aspects of the Theory of Syntax.* Cambridge, Mass.: MIT Press.

Chomsky, N. (1982). *Some Concepts and Consequences of the Theory of Government and Binding.* Cambridge, Mass.: MIT Press.

Chomsky, N. (1986). *Knowledge of Language: Its Nature, Origin, and Use.* New York: Praeger.

Chomsky, N. (2000). *New Horizons in the Study of Language and Mind.* Cambridge: Cambridge University Press.

Cicogna, C., Danesi, M., and Mollica, A. (1992) (eds.). *Problem-Solving in Second-Language Teaching.* Welland: Soleil.

Clahsen, H. (1990). The Comparative Study of First and Second Language Development. *Studies in Second Language Acquisition* 12: 135-153.

Clement, R., Gardner, R. C. and Smythe, P. C. (1980). Social and Individual Factors in Second Language Acquisition. *Canadian Journal of Behavioural Science* 12: 292-302.

Clivio, G. P. and Danesi, M. (2000). *The Sounds, Forms, and Uses of Italian: An Introduction to Italian Linguistics.* Toronto: University of Toronto Press.

Coady, J. and Huckin, T. (1977). *Second Language Vocabulary Acquisition: A Rationale for Pedagogy.* Cambridge: Canbridge University Press.

Cobley, P. (1996) (ed.). *The Communication Theory Reader.* London: Routledge.

Cohen, G. (1973). Hemispheric Differences in Serial Versus Parallel Processing. *Journal of Experimental Psychology* 97: 349-356.

Cohen, H. and Segalowitz, S. (1990). Cerebral Hemispheric Involvement in the Acquisition of New Phonetic Categories. *Brain and Language* 39: 398-409.

Cohen, N. (1984). Preserved Learning Capacity in Amnesia: Evidence for Multiple Memory Systems. In: L. R. Squire and N. Butters (eds.), *The Neuropsychology of Human Memory* 83-103. New York: Guilford.

Comrie, B. (1990). Second Language Acquisition and Language Universals Research. *Studies in Second Language Acquisition* 12: 209-218.

Connor, U. (1996). *Contrastive Rhetoric: Cross-Cultural Aspects of Second-Language Writing.* Cambridge: Cambridge University Press.

Cook, V. (1991). *Second Language Learning and Language Teaching.* London: Arnold.

Corder, S. Pit (1971). Idiosyncratic Dialects and Error Analysis. *International Review of Applied Linguistics* 9: 147-159.

Corder, S. Pit (1981). *Error Analysis and Inter-Language.* Oxford: Oxford University Press.

Cornoldi, C. and McDaniel, M. (1991). *Imagery and cognition*, Berlin: Springer.

Cotman, C. W. and Lynch, G. S. (1989). The Neurobiology of Learning and Memory. *Cognition* 33: 201-241.

Craig, C. (1986) (ed.). *Noun Classes and Categorization.* Amsterdam: John Benjamins.

Crawshaw, B. E. (1972). *Let's Play Games in French.* Skokie: National Textbook Co.

Croft, W. (1991). *Syntactic Categories and Grammatical Relations.* Chicago: University of Chicago Press.

Crookall, D. (1985) (ed.). *Simulation Applications in L2 Education and Research.* Special Issue of *System* 13, No. 3.

Crookall, D. and Oxford, R. (1988) (eds.). *Language Learning Through Simulation/Gaming.* New York: Newbury House-Harper & Row.

Crookall, D. and Saunders, D. (1989) (eds.). *Communication and Simulation: From Two Fields to One Theme.* Clevedon: Multilingual Matters.

Crookall, D., Greenblat, C., Coote, A., Klabbers, J., and Watson, D. R. (1987) (eds.). *Simulation-Gaming in the Late 1980's*. New York: Pergamon.

Cruttenden, A. (1974). An Experiment Involving Comprehension of Intonation in Children from 7 to 10. *Journal of Child Language* 1: 221-231.

Crystal, D. (1987). *The Cambridge Encyclopedia of Language*. Cambridge: Cambridge University Press.

Cummins, J. (1979). Linguistic Interdependence and the Educational Development of Bilingual Children. *Review of Educational Research* 49: 222-251.

Cummins, J. (1984). *Bilingualism and Special Education: Issues in Assessment and Pedagogy*. Clevedon: Multilingual Matters.

Cummins, J. (1986). Empowering Minority Students: A Framework for Intervention. *Harvard Educational Review* 56: 18-36.

Cummins, J. and Swain, M. (1986). *Bilingualism in Education*. London: Longman.

Curran, C. A. (1976). *Counseling-Learning in Second Languages*. Apple River, Ill.: Apple River Press.

Curro, G. (1995). A *Survey of Neurolinguistic Research and Its Implications for Second Language Teaching*. Dissertation, James Cook University of North Queensland.

Curro, G. (1995b). Neurobiology and Language Teaching. *Convivio* 1: 149-152

Curtiss, S. (1977). *Genie: A Psycholinguistic Study of a Modern-Day 'Wild Child'*. New York: Academic.

Curtiss, S. (1977). *Genie: A Psycholinguistic Study of a Modern-Day "Wild Child"*. New York: Academic.

D

D'Alfonso, A., Danesi, M., De Lellis, M., and Mastracci, M. (1986). *Problemi di neuropedagogia*. L'Aquila: Penne, Quaderni L'Ipetro 29.

D'Alonzo, L. (1993). *Handicap e potenziale educativo*. Brescia: La Scuola.

Damasio, A. R. (1994). *Descartes' Error: Emotion, Reason, and the Human Brain*. New York: G. P. Putnam's Sons.

Damasio, A. R. (1994). *Descartes' Error: Emotion, Reason, and the Human Brain*. New York: G. P. Putnam's.

Danesi, M. (1985). *A Guide to Puzzles and Games in Second Language Pedagogy*. Toronto: OISE Press.

Danesi, M. (1986). Le coordinate neurologiche dell'apprendimento linguistico: osservazioni psicopedagogiche. In: M. De Lellis (ed.), *Atti del Convegno "Il codice della mente"*, 1-24. L'Aquila: Sigma-Tau.

Danesi, M. (1988a). *Neurolinguistica e glottodidattica*. Padova: Liviana.

Danesi, M. (1988b). *Cervello, linguaggio ed educazione*. Roma: Bulzoni.

Danesi, M. (1988c). Neurological Bimodality and Theories of Language Teaching. *Studies in Second Language Acquisition* 10: 13-35.

Danesi, M. (1988d). From Context to Text: Synchronizing Language Teaching to the Neurology of Language Learning. *Die Neuren Sprachen* 87: 454-470.

Danesi, M. (1989). The Neurological Coordinates of Metaphor. *Communication & Cognition* 22: 73-86.

Danesi, M. (1990). Osservazioni neuropedagogiche sul metodo di insegnamento linguistico di "Casa Giocosa". In: M. Camuffo (ed.), *Casa Giocosa e Francesca Mineo: Quaranta anni di attività riabilitativa e di successi nel recupero psico-pedagogico e sociale del ragazzo con handicap psichico*, 85-93. Roma: Kappa.

Danesi, M. (1991). Neurological Learning Flow and Second Language Teaching: Some Evidence on the Bimodality Construct. *Rassegna Italiana di Linguistica Applicata* 23: 19-29.

Danesi, M. (1992). Metaphor and Classroom Second Language Learning. *Romance Languages Annual* 3: 189-193.

Danesi, M. (1993a). Whither Contrastive Analysis? *Canadian Modern Language Review* 50: 37-46.

Danesi, M. (1993b). Linguaggio connotativo, tono ed emozione: aspetti neuropedagogici. *Progetto Psicomotricità* 1: 84-90.

Danesi, M. (1993c). Metaphorical Competence in Second Language Acquisition and Second Language Teaching: The Neglected Dimension. In: J. E. Alatis (ed.), *Language Communication and Social Meaning*, 234-254. Washington, D. C.: Georgetown University Press.

Danesi, M. (1994a). The Neuroscientific Perspective in Second Language Acquisition Research. *International Review of Applied Linguistics* 22: 201-228.

Danesi, M. (1994b). Recent Research on Metaphor and the Teaching of Italian. *Italica* 71: 453-464.

Danesi, M. (1995). Learning and Teaching Languages: The Role of Conceptual Fluency. *International Journal of Applied Linguistics* 5: 1-12.

Danesi, M. (1999). The Dimensionality of Metaphor. *Sign Systems Studies* 27: 60-87.

Danesi, M. (2000). *Semiotics in Language Education*. Berlin: Mouton de Gruyter.

Danesi, M. and Di Pietro, R. J. (1991). *Contrastive Analysis for the Contemporary Second Language Classroom*. Toronto: OISE Press.

Danesi, M. and Mollica, A. (1988). From Right to Left: A Bimodal Perspective of Language Teaching. *Canadian Modern Language Review* 45: 76-90.

Danesi, M. and Mollica, A. M. (1998). Conceptual Fluency Theory and Second Language Teaching. *Mosaic* 5/2: 1-12.

Daniels, H. (1996) (ed.). *An Introduction to Vygotsky*. London: Routledge.

Danly, M. and Shapiro, B. (1982). Speech Prosody in Broca's Aphasia. *Brain and Language* 16: 171-190.

Davydov, V. V. and Radzikhovskii, L. A. (1985). Vygotsky's Theory and the Activity Oriented Approach in Psychology. In: J. V. Wertsch (ed.), *Culture, Communication and Cognition: Vygotskian Perspectives*, 59-69. Cambridge: Cambridge University Press.

Day, R. R. and Bamford, J. (1998). *Extensive Reading in the Second Language Classroom*. Cambridge: Cambridge Unievrsity Press.

De Lellis, M. and Cerbo, R. (1999). *Linee guida di psichiatria dello sviluppo*. Roma: Verduci.

De Villiers, J. G. and De Villiers, P. A. (1978). *Language Acquisition*. Cambridge, Mass.: Harvard University Press.

De Vries, D. L. and Slavin, R. E. (1978). Teams—Games—Tournaments: Review of Ten Classroom Experiments. *Journal of Research and Development in Education* 12: 23-38.

Deane, P. (1992). *Grammar in Mind and Brain: Explorations in Cognitive Syntax*. Berlin: Mouton de Gruyter.

Déjerine, J. (1892). Contribution à l'étude anatomo-pathologique et clinique des différents variétés de cécité verbale. *Comptes Rendus des Sciences de la Société de Biologie* 9: 61-90.

Dennis, M. and Whitaker, H. (1976). Language Acquisition following Hemidecortication: Linguistic Superiority of the Left over the Right Hemisphere. *Brain and Language* 3: 404-433.

Dewey, J. (1916). *Democracy in Education*. New York: The Free Press.

Dhority, L. (1992). *The ACT Approach: The Use of Suggestion for Integrative Learning*. New York: Gordon and Breach.

Di Pietro, R. J. (1971). *Language Structures in Contrast*. Rowley, Mass.: Newbury House.

Di Pietro, R. J. (1987). *Strategic Interaction*. Cambridge: Cambridge University Press.

Diadori, P. (1990). *Senza parole: 100 gesti degli italiani*. Roma: Bonacci.

Dickson, P. S. (1992). Quick and Easy Games for Language Learning. In: C. Cicogna, M. Danesi, and A. Mollica (eds.), *Problem-Solving in Second-Language Teaching*, 223-241. Welland: Soleil.

Diller, K. (1978). *The Language Teaching Controversy*. Rowley Mass.: Newbury House Publishers.

Dimitrijevic, N. (1977). Applied Neurolinguistics: One Step Nearer the Formulation of a Model for Foreign Language Learning. *Studi Italiani di Linguistica Teorica ed Applicata* 9: 235-260.

Dirven, R. and Verspoor, M. (1998). *Cognitive Exploration of Language and Linguistics*. Amsterdam: John Benjamins.

Doggett, G. (1994). Eight Approaches to Language Teaching. *Mosaic* 1: 8-12.

Doughty, C. and Williams, J. (1998). *Focus on Form in Classroom Second Language Acquisition*. New York: Cambridge University Press.

Dulay, H., Burt, M. K., and Krashen, S. (1982). *Language Two*. Oxford: Oxford University Press.

Dunn, B. R. (1985). Bimodal Processing and Memory from Text. In: V. M. Rentel, S. A. Corson, and B. R. Dunn (eds.), *Psychophysiological Aspects of Reading and Learning*, 12-29. New York: Gordon and Breach.

Dusková, L. (1969). On Sources of Errors in Foreign Language Learning. *International Review of Applied Linguistics* 7: 11-36.

E

Edwards, B. (1979). *Drawing on the Right Side of the Brain*. Los Angeles: J. P. Tarcher.

Edwards, D. (1997). *Discourse and Cognition*. London: Sage.

Ehrman, M. E. (1996). *Understanding Second Language Learning Difficulties*. Thousand Oaks, Ca.: Sage Publications.

Eimas P. D. and Galaburda, A. M. (1989)., Some Agenda Items for a Neurobiology of Cognition: An Introduction *Cognition* 33: 1-23.

Elliott, A. R. (1995). Filed Independence/Dependence, Hemispheric Specialization, and Attitude in Relation to Pronunciation Accuracy in Spanish as a Foreign Language. *Modern Language Journal* 79: 356-371.

Ellis, N. (1994). *Implicit and Explicit Learning of Languages*. New York: Academic Press.

Ellis, R. (1997). *Second Language Acquisition*. Oxford: Oxford University Press.

Entwistle, W. (1981). *Styles of Learning and Teaching*. New York: John Wiley.

Ervin Tripp, S. M. and Slobin, D. I. (1966). Psycholinguistics. *Annual Review of Psychology* 17: 435.

Ervin, G. L. (1982). Using Warm-Ups, Wind-Ups, and Fillers: *All* of Your Class Time is Valuable. *Foreign Language Annals* 15: 95-99.

Eubank, L. (1991) (ed.). *Point Counterpoint: Universal Grammar in the Second Language*. Amsterdam: John Benjamins.

Eubank, L. and Gregg, K. R. (1995). Et in Amygdala Ego? UG, (S)LA, and Neurobiology. *Studies in Second Language Acquisition* 17: 35-57.

Extra, G. and Verhoeven, L. (1999) (eds.). *Bilingualism and Migration*. Berlin: Mouton de Gruyter.

F

Fabbro, F. (1990). Cerebral Lateralization in Simultaneous Interpretation. *Brain and Language* 39: 69-89.

Fabbro, F. (1999). *The Neurolinguistics of Bilingualism: An Introduction*. Hove: Psychology Press.

Fabbro, F., Gran, B., and Gran, L. (1991). Hemispheric Specialization for Semantic and Syntactic Comprehension of Language in Simultaneous Interpretation. *Brain and Language* 41: 1-42.

Faerch, C., Haastrup, K., and Phillipson, R. (1984). *Learner Language and Language Learning*. Clevedon: Multilingual Matters.

Fass, D. (1997). *Processing Metonymy and Metaphor*. Greenwich, Conn.: Ablex Publishing.

Fauconnier, G. (1985). *Mental Spaces*. Cambridge: Cambridge University Press.

Fauconnier, G. (1997). *Mappings in Thought and Language*. Cambridge: Cambridge University Press.

Fauconnier, G. and Sweetser, E. (1996) (eds.). *Spaces, Worlds, and Grammar*. Chicago: University of Chicago Press.

Fauconnier, G. and Turner, M. (2002). The Way We Think: Conceptual Blending and the Mind's Hidden Complexities. New York: Basic.

Faust, M., Kravitz, S., and Babkoff, H. (1993a). Hemisphericity and Top-Down Processing of Language. *Brain and Language* 44: 1-18.

Faust, M., Kravitz, S., and Babkoff, H. (1993b). Hemispheric Specialization for Reading Habits: Evidence from Lexical Decision Research with Hebrew Words and Sentences. *Brain and Language* 44: 254-263.

Feez, S. (1998). *Text-Based Syllabus Design*. New South Wales: Ames.

Felder, R. M. and Henriques, E. R. (1995). Learning and Teaching Styles in Foreign and Second Language Education. *Foreign Language Annals* 28: 21-31.

Firth, J. R. (1957). *Papers in Linguistics: 1934-1951*. Oxford: Oxford University Press.

Fisiak, J. (1981) (ed.). *Contrastive Analysis and the Language Teacher*. Oxford: Pergamon Press.

Flege, J. L. (1987). A Critical Period for Learning to Pronounce Foreign Languages? *Applied Linguistics* 8: 162-177.

Fries, C. F. (1927). *The Teaching of the English Language*. New York: Appleton Century.

Fries, C. F. (1945). *Teaching and Learning English as a Foreign Language*. Ann Arbor: University of Michigan Press.

G

Gall, F. J. (1791). *Philosophisch-medicinische Untersuchungen*. Vienna: Gräffer.

Galloway, L. M. (1983). The Convolutions of Second Language: A Theoretical Article with a Critical Review and Some New Hypotheses towards a Neuropsychological Model of Bilingualism and Second Language Performance. *Language Learning* 31: 439-463.

Galloway, L. M. and Krashen, S. D. (1980). Cerebral Organization in Bilingualism and Second Language. In: R. C. Scarcella and S. D. Krashen (eds.), *Research in Second Language Acquisition*, 74-80. Rowley, Mass.: Newbury House.

Garau, P. (1992). The Competent English Teacher and the Triune Brain. *Perspectives* 18: 65-69.

Gardner, H. (1982). *Art, Mind, and Brain: A Cognitive Approach to Creativity*. New York: Basic.

Gardner, H. (1983). *Frames of Mind: The Theory of Multiple Intelligences*. New York: Basic.

Gardner, H., Winner, E., Bechofer, R., and Wolf, D. (1978). The Development of Figurative Language. In: K. Nelson (ed.), *Children's Language*, 1-38. New York: Garner Press.

Garrett, N. (1986). The Problem with Grammar: What Kind Can the Language Learner Use? *Modern Language Journal* 70: 133-148.

Gass, S. (1983). The Development of L2 Intuitions. *TESOL Quarterly* 17: 273-291.

Gass, S. and Madden, C. (1985) (eds.). *Input in Second Language Acquisition*. Rowley, Mass.: Newbury House.

Gass, S. and Selinker, L. (1994). *Second Language Acquisition: An Introductory Course*. Hillsdale: Lawrence Erlbaum Associates.

Gass, S. M. and Houk, N. (1999). *Interlanguage Refusals: A Cross-Cultural Study of Japanese English*. Berlin: Mouton de Gruyter.

Gattegno, C. (1972). *Teaching Foreign Languages in Schools: The Silent Way*. New York: Education Solutions.

Gattegno, C. (1976). *The Common Sense of Teaching Foreign Languages*. New York: Educational Solutions.

Gattegno, C. (1976). *The Common Sense of Teaching Foreign Languages*. New York: Educational Solutions.

Gazzaniga, M. (1988). *The Social Mind: Discovering the Networks of the Mind*. New York: Basic.

Gazzaniga, M. S. (1973). *Fundamentals of Psychology*. New York: Academic.

Gazzaniga, M. S. and Sperry, R. W. (1967). Language after Section of the Cerebral Commissures. *Brain* 90: 131-148.

Gazzaniga, M. S., Bogen, J. E., and Sperry, R. W. (1963). Laterality Effects in Somesthesis following Cerebral Commissurotomy in Man. *Neuropsychologia* 1: 209-215.

Genesee, F. (1982). Experimental Neuropsychological Research on Second Language Processing. *TESOL Quarterly* 16: 315-324.

Genesee, F. (1987). *Learning through Two Languages*. Rowley, Mass.: Newbury House.

Genesee, F. (1988). Neuropsychology and Second Language Acquisition. In: L. M. Beebe (ed.), *Issues in Second Language Acquisition: Multiple Perspectives*, 81-112. Rowley, Mass.: Newbury House.

Gerrig R. and Healey, A. (1983). Dual Processes in Metaphor Understanding: Comprehension and Appreciation. *Journal of Experimental Psychology: Learning, Memory, and Cognition* 9: 667-675.

Geschwind, N. and Galaburda, A. (1987). *Cerebral Lateralization: Biological Mechanisms, Associations, and Pathology*. Cambridge, Mass.: MIT Press.

Gibbs, R. W. (1994). *The Poetics of Mind: Figurative Thought, Language, and Understanding*. Cambridge: Cambridge University Press.

Goatley, A. (1997). *The Language of Metaphors*. London: Routledge.

Goldberg, E. and Costa, L. D. (1981). Hemispheric Differences in the Acquisition of Descriptive Systems. *Brain and Language* 14: 144-173.

Gouin, F. (1880). *L'art d'enseigner et d'étudier les langues*. Paris: Librairie Fischbacher.

Grabe, W. (1991). Current Developments in Second Language Reading Research. *TESOL Quarterly* 25: 375-406.

Green, A., Nicholson, N. S., Vaid, J., and White, A. (1990). Hemispheric Involvement in Shadowing vs. Interpretation: A Time-Sharing Study of Simultaneous Interpretation with Matched Bilingual and Monolingual Controls. *Brain and Language* 39: 107-133.

Gregg, K. (1984). Krashen's Monitor and Occam's Razor. *Applied Linguistics* 5: 79-100.

Grosjean, F. (1989). Neurolinguists Beware! The Bilingual Is Not Two Monolinguals in One Person. *Brain and Language* 36: 3-15.

H

Hachinski, K. V. and Hachinski, V. (1994). Music and the Brain. *Canadian Medical Association Journal* 151: 293-295.

Haden Elgin, S. (2000). *The Language Imperative*. Cambridge, Mass.: Perseus.

Hakuta, K. (1986). *Mirror of Language: The Debate on Bilingualism*. New York: Basic Books.

Hall, E. T. (1966). *The Hidden Dimension*. New York: Doubleday.

Halliday, M. A. K. (1973). *Explorations in the Functions of Language*. London: Edward Arnold.

Halliday, M. A. K. (1975). *Learning How to Mean: Explorations in the Development of Language*. London: Arnold.

Halliday, M. A. K. (1985). *Introduction to Functional Grammar*. London: Arnold.

Halliday, M. A. K., McIntosh, A., and Strevens, P. (1964). *The Linguistic Sciences and Language Teaching*. London: Longman.

Hamers, J. F. and Blanc, M. H. A. (1989). *Bilinguality and Bilingualism* Cambridge: Cambridge University Press.

Hamers, J. T. and Lambert, W. E. (1977). Visual Field and Cerebral Hemispheric Preferences: In: S. J. Segalowitz and F. A. Gruber (eds.), *Bilinguals in Language Development and Neurological Theories of Language*. New York: Academic.

Hammerly, H. (1995). What Visual Aids Can and Cannot Do in Second Language Teaching. *Mosaic* 2: 11-17.

Hardyck, C. (1977). A Model of Individual Differences in Hemispheric Functioning. In: H. .A. Whitaker (ed.), *Studies in Neurolinguistics,* 223-255. New York: Academic Press.

Harley, B. (1986). *Age in Second Language Acquisition.* Clevedon: Multilingual Matters Ltd.

Heilman, K. M., Scholes, R., and Watson, R. T. (1975). Auditory Affective Agnosia: Disturbed Comprehension of Affective Speech. *Journal of Neurology, Neurosurgery and Psychiatry* 38: 69-72.

Hendrickson, J. M. (1980). Listening and Speaking Activities for Foreign Language Learners. *Canadian Modern Language Review* 36: 735-748.

Hendrickson, J. M. (1983). Listening and Speaking Activities for Foreign Language Learners: Second Collection. *Canadian Modern Language Review* 39: 267-284.

Henry, A. R. (1993). *Second Language Rhetorics in Process: A Comparison of Arabic, Chinese, and Spanish.* New York: Peter Lang.

Hermann, N. (1988). *The Creative Brain.* Lake Lure, N. C.: Brain Books.

Herschensohn, J. (1990). Towards a Theoretical Basis for Current Language Pedagogy. *Modern Language Journal* 74: 450-458.

Hickok, G., Bellugi, U., and Klima, E. S. (2001). Sign Language in the Brain. *Scientific American* 284/6: 58-65.

Hier, D. B. and Kaplan, J. (1980). Verbal Comprehension Deficits after Right Hemisphere Damage. *Applied Psycholinguistics* 1: 270-294.

Hinkel, E. (1999). *Culture in Second Language Teaching and Learning.* Cambridge: Cambridge University Press.

Holden, C. (1994). Random Samples: Smart Music. *Science* 266: 968-969.

Honeck, R. P. and Hoffman, R. (1980) (eds.). *Cognition and Figurative Language.* Hillsdale, N. J.: Lawrence Erlbaum.

Honeck, R. P. and Hoffman, R. P. (198) (eds.). *Cognition and Figurative Language.* Hillsdale, N. J.: Lawrence Erlbaum.

Hough, M. S. (1990). Narrative Comprehension in Adults with Right and Left Hemisphere Brain Damage: Theme Organization. *Brain and Language* 38: 253-277.

House, J. (1996). Developing Pragmatic Fluency in English as a Foreign Language: Routines and Metapragmatic Awareness. *Studies in Second Language Acquisition* 18: 225-252.

Hunter, N. and Liederman, J. (1991). Right Hemisphere Participation in Reading. *Brain and Language* 41: 475-495.

Hupb, L. B. (1974). *Let's Play Games in Spanish.* Skokie: National Textbook Co.

Hurford, J. R. (1991). The Evolution of a Critical Period for Language Acquisition. *Cognition* 40: 159-201.

Hutchby, I. and Wooffitt, R. (1998). *Conversation Analysis.* Cambridge: Polity Press.

Hyltenstam, K. and Obler, L. (1987) (eds.). *Bilingualism across the Lifespan: Aspects of Acquisition, Maturity, and Loss.* Cambridge: Cambridge University Press.

Hymes, D. (1971). *On Communicative Competence.* Philadelphia: University of Pennsylvania Press.

Hymes, D. (1972). On Communicative Competence. In: J. B. Pride and J. Holmes (eds.), *Sociolinguistics: Selected Readings*, 269-293. Harmondsworth: Penguin.

I

In

durkhya, B. (1992). *Metaphor and Cognition.* Dordrecht: Kluwer.

Ingram, D. (1989). *First Language Acquisition: Method, Description, and Explanation.* Cambridge: Cambridge University Press.

Ingram, D. (1989). *First Language Acquisition: Method, Description, and Explanation.* Cambridge: Cambridge University Press.

Inhelder, B. and Piaget, J. (1958). *The Growth of Logical Thinking from Childhood through Adolescence.* New York: Basic.

Irwing, P. (1982). Games for Use at the Intermediate Level. *Canadian Modern Language Review* 38: 726-727.

J

Jackson, J. H. (1874). On the Nature and Duality of the Brain. *Medical Press and Circular* 1: 19-41.

Jackson, J. H. (1878). On Affectives of Speech from Disease of the Brain. *Brain* 1: 304-330.

Jacobs, B. (1988). Neurobiological Differentiation of Primary and Secondary Language Acquisition. *Studies in Second Language Acquisition* 10: 303-337.

Jacobs, B. (1995). Dis-Integrating Perspectives of Language Acquisition: A Response to Eubank and Gregg. *Studies in Second Language Acquisition* 17: 65-72.

Jacobs, B. and Schumann, J. (1992). Language Acquisition and the Neurosciences: Towards a More Integrative Perspective. *Applied Linguistics* 13: 282-301.

Jakobovits, L. A. (1970). *Foreign Language Learning: A Psycholinguistic Analysis of the Issues.* Rowley, Mass.: Newbury House.

Jakobson, R. (1942). *Kindersprache, Aphasie und algemeine Lautgesetze.* Uppsala: Almqvist and Wiksell.

Jakobson, R. (1960). Linguistics and Poetics. In: T. A. Sebeok (ed.), *Style and Language*, 34-45. Cambridge, Mass.: MIT Press.

James, C. (1980). *Contrastive Analysis.* London: Longman.

Janssen, T. and Redeker, G. (1999) (eds.). *Cognitive Linguistics: Foundations, Scope, and Methodology.* Berlin: Mouton de Gruyter.

Jay, T. (1999). *Why We Curse: A Neuro-Psycho-Social Theory of Speech.* Amsterdam: John Benjamins.

Jeffries, S. (1985). English Grammar Terminology as an Obstacle to Second Language Learning. *Modern Language Journal* 69: 385-390.

Jesperson, O. (1904). *How to Teach a Foreign Language.* London: Allen and Unwin.

Joanette, Y. and Goulet, P. (1988). Word Naming in Right-Brain Damaged Patients. In: C. Chiarello (ed.), *Right Hemisphere Contributions to Lexical Semantics*, 1-18. Berlin: Springer Verlag.

Joanette, Y., Goulet, P., and Hannequin, D. (1990) (eds.). *Right Hemisphere and Verbal Communication.* Berlin: Springer.

Johnson, J. and Rosano, T. (1993). Relation of Cognitive Style to Metaphor Interpretation and Second Language Proficiency. *Applied Psycholinguistics* 14: 159-175.

Johnson, J. S. and Newport, E. L. (1989). Critical Period Effects in Second Language Learning: The Influence of Maturational State on the Acquisition of English as a Second Language. *Cognitive Psychology* 21: 60-99.

Johnson, J. S. and Newport, E. L. (1991). Critical Period Effects on Universal Properties of Language: The Status of Subjacency in the Acquisition of a Second Language. *Cognition* 39: 215-258.

Johnson, K. (1996.). *Language Teaching & Skill Learning.* Oxford: Blackwell.

Johnson, M. (1987). *The Body in the Mind: The Bodily Basis of Meaning, Imagination, and Reason.* Chicago: University of Chicago Press.

Johnson, S. (1979). *Nonverbal Communication in the Teaching of Foreign Languages.* Dissertation, Indiana University.

Johnson-Weiner, K. M. (1984). The Effects of Right and Left Hemisphere Damage on the Comprehension of Stress in English. In: A. Manning, P. Martin, and K. McCalla (eds.), *The Tenth LACUS Forum*, 464-473. Columbia, S. C.: Hornbeam.

Jones, K. (1982). *Simulations in Language Teaching*. Cambridge: Cambridge University Press.

Jones, K. (1986). *Designing Your Own Simulations*. New York: Methuen.

Jones, R. (1982). *Physics as Metaphor*. New York: New American Library.

Joos, M. (1967). *The Five Clocks*. New York: Harcourt, Brace and World.

Joseph, R. (1992). *The Right Brain and the Unconscious: Discovering the Stranger Within*. New York: Plenum.

Joynt R. J. (1964). Paul Pierre Broca: His Contribution to the Knowledge of Aphasia. *Cortex* 2: 206-213.

K

Kandel, E. R., Schwartz, J. H., and Jessell, T. M. (1991). *Principles of Neuroscience*. New York: Elsevier.

Kaplan, J. A., Brownell, H. H., Jacobs, J. R. and Gardner, H. (1990). The Effects of Right Hemisphere Damage on the Pragmatic Interpretation of Conversational Remarks. *Brain and Language* 38: 315-333.

Kaplan, R. D. (1966). Cultural Thought Patterns in Inter-Cultural Education. *Language Learning* 16: 1-20.

Kaplan, R. D. (1978). Contrastive Rhetoric: Some Hypotheses. *Review of Applied Linguistics* 39: 61-72.

Katona, G. (1940). *Organizing and Memorizing: Studies in the Psychology of Learning and Teaching*. New York: Columbia University Press

Kelly, L. G. (1969). *25 Centuries of Language Teaching*. Rowley, Mass.: Newbury House.

Kimura, D. (1963). Speech Lateralization in Young Children as Determined by an Auditory Test. *Journal of Comparative and Physiological Psychology*. 56: 899-902.

Kimura, D. (1993). *Neuromotor Mechanisms in Human Communication*. New York: Oxford Unievrsity Press.

Kinsbourne, M. and Hicock, M. (1977). Does Cerebral Dominance Develop?. In: J. Segalowitz and F. A. Gruber, *Language Development and Neurological Theory*, 171-191. New York: Academic.

Kosslyn, S. M. (1983). *Ghosts in the Mind's Machine: Creating and Using Images in the Brain*. New York: W. W. Norton.

Kotulak, R. (1996). *Inside the Brain: Revolutionary Discoveries of How the Mind Works*. Kansas City: Andrews and McMeel.

Kövecses, Z. (1986). *Metaphors of Anger, Pride, and Love: A Lexical Approach to the Structure of Concepts*. Amsterdam: John Benjamins.

Kövecses, Z. (1988). *The Language of Love: The Semantics of Passion in Conversational English*. London: Associated University Presses.

Kövecses, Z. (1990). *Emotion Concepts*. New York: Springer.

Krampen, M. (1991). *Children's Drawings: Iconic Coding of the Environment*. New York: Plenum.

Kramsch, C. (1998). *Language and Culture*. Oxford: Oxford University Press.

Krashen, S. D. (1973). Lateralization, Language Learning and the Critical Period: Some New Evidence. *Language Learning* 23: 63-74.

Krashen, S. D. (1975). The Development of Cerebral Dominance and Language Learning: More New Evidence. In: D. Dato (ed.), *Developmental Psycholinguistics*, 179-192. Washington, D. C.: Georgetown University Press.

Krashen, S. D. (1982). *Principles and Practice in Second Language Acquisition*. Oxford: Pergamon.

Krashen, S. D. (1985). *The Input Hypothesis*. London : Longman.

Krashen, S. D. (1991). *Bilingual Education: A Focus on Current Research*. Washington, D. C.: National Clearinghouse for Bilingual Education.

Krashen, S. D. and Terrell, T. (1983). *The Natural Approach: Language Acquisition in the Classroom.* Oxford: Pergamon.

Kress, G. (1985). *Linguistic Processes in Sociocultural Practice.* Melbourne: Deakin University Press.

Kress, G. (1995). *Making Signs and Making Subjects: The English Curriculum and Social Futures.* London: Institute of Education.

Kroll, B. (1990) (ed.). *Second Language Writing: Research Insight for the Classroom.* Cambridge: Cambridge University Press.

Kufner, H. L. (1962). *The Grammatical Structures of English and German.* Chicago: University of Chicago Press.

Kuhn, T. S. (1970). *The Structure of Scientific Revolutions.* Chicago: University of Chicago Press.

L

Lado, R. (1957). *Linguistics Across Cultures: Applied Linguistics for Language Teachers.* Ann Arbor: University of Michigan Press.

Lado, R. (1964). *Language Teaching: A Scientific Approach.* New York: McGraw-Hill.

Ladousse, G. P. (1987). *Role Play.* Oxford: Oxford University Press.

Lakoff, G. (1987). *Women, Fire, and Dangerous Things: What Categories Reveal about the Mind.* Chicago: University of Chicago Press.

Lakoff, G. and Johnson, M. (1980). *Metaphors We Live By.* Chicago: Chicago University Press.

Lakoff, G. and Johnson, M. (1999). *Philosophy in the Flesh.* New York: Basic.

Lakoff, G. and Turner, M. (1989). *More than Cool Reason: A Field Guide to Poetic Metaphor.* Chicago: University of Chicago Press.

Lamb, S. M. (1999). *Pathways of the Brain: The Neurocognitive Basis of Language.* Amsterdam: John Benjamins.

Lamendella, J. T. (1977a). The Limbic System in Human Communication. In: H. A. Whitaker (ed.), *Studies in Neurolinguistics*, 157-222. New York: Academic.

Lamendella, J. T. (1977b). General Principles of Neurofunctional Organization and Their Manifestation in Primary and Non-Primary Acquisition. *Language Learning* 27: 155-196.

Lamendella, J. T. (1979). The Neurofunctional Basis of Pattern Practice. *TESOL Quarterly* 13: 5-19.

Langacker, R. W. (1987). *Foundations of Cognitive Grammar.* Stanford: Stanford University Press.

Langacker, R. W. (1990). *Concept, Image, and Symbol: The Cognitive Basis of Grammar.* Berlin: Mouton de Gruyter.

Langacker, R. W. (1999). *Grammar and Conceptualization.* Berlin: Mouton de Gruyter.

Langer, S. K. (1948). *Philosophy in a New Key.* Cambridge: Harvard University Press.

Larsen-Freeman, D. (1986). *Techniques and Principles in Language Teaching.* Oxford: Oxford University Press.

Lashley, K. S. (1929). *Brain Mechanisms and Intelligence.* Chicago: University of Chicago Press.

Latorre, G. and Baeza, G. (1975). The Construction and Use of EFL Crossword Puzzles. *English Language Teaching Journal* 30: 45-55.

Lattey, E. (1986). Pragmatic Classification of Idioms as an Aid for the Language Learner. *International Review of Applied Linguistics* 24: 217-233.

Lautrey, J. D. and Chartier, A. (1991). A Developmental Approach to Mental Imagery. In: C. Cornoldi and M. A. McDaniel (eds.), *Imagery and Cognition*, 248-282. New York: Springer.

Lebrun, Y. (1977). Neurolinguistic Models of Language and Speech. In: H. A. Whitaker (ed.), *Studies in Neurolinguistics*, 1-29. New York: Academic.

Lee, W. R. (1965). *Language Teaching Games and Contests.* Oxford: Oxford University Press.

Leezenberg, M. (2001). Contexts of Metaphor. Amsterdam: Elsevier

Leki, I. (1991). Twenty-Five Years of Contrastive Rhetoric: Text Analysis and Writing Pedagogies. *TESOL Quarterly* 25: 123-143.

Lenneberg, E. (1967). *The Biological Foundations of Language.* New York: John Wiley.

Lepschy, G. (1994). *History of Linguistics.* London: Longman.

Lesgold, A. (1988). Problem Solving. In: R. J. Sternberg and E. E. Smith (eds.), *The Psychology of Human Thought*, 188-213. Cambridge: Cambridge University Press.

Levelt, W. J. M. (1992). Psycholinguistics. An Overview. In: W. Bright (ed.), *International Encyclopedia of Linguistics*, vol. 3, 290-294. Oxford, Oxford University Press.

Levin, S. (1977). *The Semantics of Metaphor.* Baltimore: Johns Hopkins Press.

Levy, J., Trevarthen, C., and Sperry, R. W. (1972). Perception of Bilateral Chimeric Figures following Hemispheric Disconnection. *Brain* 95: 61-78.

Lewandowsky, S., Dunn, J. C. and Kirsner, K. (1989) (eds.). *Implicit Memory: Theoretical Issues.* Hillsdale, N. J.: Lawrence Erlbaum Associates.

Lewis, M. (1993). *The Lexical Approach.* Hove: Language Teaching Publications.

Lewis, M. (1997). *Implementing the Lexical Approach: Putting Theory into Practice.* Hove: Language Teaching Publications.

Lieberman, P. (2000). *Human Language and Our Reptilian Brain.* Cambridge, Mass.: Harvard University Press.

Livingston, S. A. and Kidder, S. J. (1973). Role Identification and Game Structure: Effects on Political Attitudes. *Simulation and Games* 4: 131-144.

Loftus, G. R. and Loftus, E. F. (1983). *Mind at Play.* New York: Basic Books.

Logie, R. H. (1991). Visuo-Spatial Short-Term Memory: Visual Working Memory or Visual Buffer? In: C. Cornoldi and M. A. McDaniel (eds.), *Imagery and Cognition*, 77-102. New York: Springer.

Lombardo, L. (1988). Helping Learners to Establish Criteria in an L2: Promoting Learner Autonomy in the Foreign Language Classroom. In: G. Cecioni (ed.), *Proceedings of the Symposium on Autonomy in Foreign Language Learning*, 70-79. Firenze: Centro Linguistico di Ateneo.

Long, M. H. (1995). The Least a Second Language Acquisition Theory Needs to Explain. In: H. Douglas Brown and S. Gonzo (eds.), *Readings on Second Language Acquisition*, 470-490. Englewood Cliffs: Prentice Hall.

Long, M. H. (1995). The Least a Second Language Acquisition Theory Needs to Explain. In: H. D. Brown and S. Gonzo (eds.), *Readings on Second Language Acquisition*, 470-490. Englewood Cliffs, NJ: Prentice Hall.

Lozanov, G, (1979). *Suggestology and Outline of Suggestopedy.* New York: Gordon and Breach.

Ludwig, J. M. (1979). The Cognitive Method and Error Analysis. *Foreign Language Annals* 12: 209-212.

Lugton, R. (1971) (eds.). *Toward a Cognitive Approach to Second Language Acquisition.* Philadelphia: Center for Curriculum Development.

Luria, A. R. (1947). *Traumatic Aphasia.* The Hague: Mouton.

Luria, A. R. (1974a). Basic Problems of Neurolinguistics. In: T. A. Sebeok (ed.), *Current Trends in Linguistics*, vol. 12, 2516-2594. The Hague: Mouton.

Luria, A. R. (1974b). Language and Brain: Towards the Basic Problems of Neurolinguistics. *Brain and Language* 1: 1-14.

M

MacLaury, R. E. (1997). *Color and Cognition in Mesoamerica: Constructing Categories as Vantages.* Austin: University of Texas Press.

MacLennan, C. H. G. (1994). Metaphors and Prototypes in the Learning and Teaching of Grammar and Vocabulary. *International Review of Applied Linguistics* 32: 97-110.

MacWhinney, B. (2000). Connectionism and Language Learning. In: M. Barlow and S. Kemmer (eds.), *Usage Models of Language*, pp.121-150. Stanford: Center for the Study of Language and Information.

Magnan, S. S. (1988). Grammar and the ACTFL Oral Proficiency Interview: Discussion and Data. *Modern Language Journal* 72: 266-276.

Maiguascha, R. (1984). Semantic Fields: Towards a Methodology for Teaching Vocabulary in the L2 Classroom. *Canadian Modern Language Review* 40: 274-97.

Maiguascha, R. (1984). Semantic Fields: Towards a Methodology for Teaching Vocabulary in the L2 Classroom. *Canadian Modern Language Review* 40: 274-97.

Maiguascha, R. (1989). Il linguaggio figurato nella didattica dell'italiano come lingua seconda: una proposta metodologica. In: A. N. Mancini and P. Giordano (eds.), *Italiana 1987*, 36-35. River Forest: Rosary College.

Maiguascha, R. (1993). A Robin is More of a Bird than a Penguin: Prototype Theory and the Teaching of Vocabulary. In: V. Adamantova, L. G. Sbrocchi, and R. Williamson (eds.), 112-127. *L2 and Beyond: Teaching and Learning Modern Languages*. Ottawa: Legas Publishing.

Maiguashca, R. (1988). Quanto "valgono" le parole straniere? *Italiano e Oltre* 3: 136-139.

Maley, A. and Grellet, F. (1981). *Mind Matters*. Cambridge: Cambridge University Press.

Martin, O. S. (1982). Brain and Language: The Rules of the Game. In: M. A. Arbib, D. Caplan and J. C. Marshall (eds.), *Neural Models of Language Processes*, 23-36. New York: Academic Press.

Marton, W. (1974). Syllabus Design and the Cognitive Approach to Foreign-Language Teaching. *ITL: Review of Applied Linguistics* 25-26: 19-34.

Masella, A. B. and Portner, I. A. (1981). "Body Language" in Italian. *Italica* 58: 205-213.

Matsuda, P. K. (1997). Contrastive Rhetoric in Context: A Dynamic Model of L2 Writing. *Journal of Second Language Writing* 6: 45-60.

McArthur, T. (1984). *A Foundation Course for Language Teachers*. Cambridge: Cambridge University Press.

McCafferty, S. G. (1994). Adult Second Language Learners' Use of Private Speech: A Review of Studies. *Modern Language Journal* 78: 4210436.

McKay, S. L. (1980). On Notional Syllabuses. *Modern Language Journal* 64: 179-186.

McKay, S. L. (1985). *Teaching Grammar*. Oxford: Pergamon.

McKeener, W. W. and Hunt, L. J. (1989). Language Laterality in Navajo Reservation Children: Dichotic Tests Results Depend on the Language Context of the Testing. *Brain and Language* 36: 148-158.

McLaughlin, B. (1987). *Theories of Second-Language Learning*. London: Edward Arnold.

McNeill, D. (1966). The Creation of Language. *Discovery* 37: 34-38.

McNeill, D. (1987). *Psycholinguistics: A New Approach*. New York: Harper and Row.

McNeill, D. (1992). *Hand and Mind: What Gestures Reveal about Thought*. Chicago: University of Chicago Press.

Mendelsohn, S. (1988). Language Lateralization in Bilinguals: Facts and Fantasy. *Journal of Neuroscience* 3: 261-292.

Mignault, L. B. (1978). Suggestopedia: Is There a Better Way to Learn? *Canadian Modern Language Review* 34: 695-701.

Milberg, W. (1988). Representation, Control and Interaction: What Would a Theory of Right-Hemisphere Lexical Semantics Look Like? In: C. Chiarello (ed.), *Right Hemisphere Contributions to Lexical Semantics*, 89-98. New York: Springer.

Miller, G. A. (1956). The Magical Number Seven Plus or Minus Two: Some Limits to Our Capacity for Processing Information. *Psychological Review* 6: 81-97.

Miller, G. A. (1978) (ed.). *Psychology and Biology of Language and Thought. Essays in Honor of Eric Lenneberg.*, New York: Academic.

Miller, G. A. and Gildea, P. M. (1991). How Children Learn Words. In: S-Y Wand (ed.), *The Emergence of Language: Development and Evolution*, 150-158. New York: W. H. Freeman.

Miller, M. C. (1992). *Two Experimental Studies of the Effectiveness of Interactive Game-Playing in the Acquisition of Japanese by American Students*. Dissertation, University of Delaware.

Mitchell, M. (1993). *Analogy-Making as Perception: A Computer Model*. Cambridge, Mass.: MIT Press.

Mitchell, R. and Myles, F. (1998). *Second Language Learning Theories*. New York: Cambridge University Press.

Mohan, B. A. (1986). *Language and Content*. Reading, Mass.: Addison-Wesley.

Mollica, A. (1979). Games and Activities in the Italian High School Classroom. *Foreign Language Annals* 12: 347-354.

Mollica, A. (1981). Visual Puzzles in the Second Language Classroom. *Canadian Modern Language Review* 37: 583-622.

Mollica, A. (1991). *Parole crociate per principianti*. Welland: Soleil.

Mollica, A. (1992). Reinforcing Language Skills through Problem-Solving and Pencil and Paper Activities. In: C. Cicogna, M. Danesi, and A. Mollica (eds.), *Problem-Solving in Second-Language Teaching*, 102-129. Welland: Soleil.

Morris, C. (1938). *Foundations of the Theory of Signs*. Chicago: University of Chicago Press.

Morris, C. (1946). *Writings on the General Theory of Signs*. The Hague: Mouton.

Morris, D. (1979). *Gestures: Their Origins and Distributions*. London: Cape.

Musumeci, D. (1992). Selecting Games for the Second-Language Classroom: Criteria for Multiple Functions. In: C. Cicogna, M. Danesi, and A. Mollica (eds.), *Problem-Solving in Second-Language Teaching*, 242-253. Welland: Soleil.

Musumeci, D. (1997). *Breaking Tradition: An Exploration of the Historical Relationship between Theory and Practice in Second Language Teaching*. New York: McGraw-Hill.

Myers, R. E. and Sperry, R. W. (1958). Interhemispheric Communication through the Corpus Callosum: Mnemonic Carry-Over between the Hemispheres. *Archives of Neurology and Psychiatry* 80: 298-303.

N

Nation, I. S. P. (1990). *Teaching and Learning Vocabulary*. Boston: Heinle and Heinle.

Neisser, U. (1987) (ed.). *Concepts and Conceptual Development: Ecological and Intellectual Factors in Categorization*. Cambridge: Cambridge University Press.

Nelson, K. (1996). *Language in Cognitive Development: The Emergence of the Mediated Mind*. Cambridge: Cambridge University Press.

Nemser, W. (1971). Approximative Systems of Foreign Language Learners. *International Review of Applied Linguistics* 9: 115-123.

Newmark, L. and Reibel, B. (1966). Necessity and Sufficiency in Language Learning. *International Review of Applied Linguistics* 40: 157-165.

Nuessel, F. (1994). Recreational Problem-Solving Activities for Teaching Vocabulary and Intermediate Spanish. *Hispania* 77: 118-124.

Nuessel, F. (1994). Recreational problem-Solving Activities for Teaching Vocabulary in Elementary and Intermediate Spanish. *Hispania* 77: 118-124.

Nuessel, F. and Cicogna, C. (1992). Pedagogical Applications of the Bimodal Model of Learning through Visual and Auditory Stimuli. *Romance Languages Annual* 3: 289-292.

Nuessel, F. and Cicogna, C. (1993). Narrative Texts and Images in the Teaching of the Italian Language and Italian Culture. *Romance Languages Annual* 4: 319-324.

Nunan, D. (1988). *Syllabus Design*. Oxford: Oxford University Press.

Nunan, D. (1991). *Language Teaching Methodology: A textbook for Teachers*. New York: Prentice-Hall.

Nuttall, C. (1996). *Teaching Reading Skills in a Foreign Language*. Oxford: Heinemann.

Nuyts, J. (2001). *Epistemic Modality, Language, and Conceptualization: A Cognitive-Pragmatic Perspective*. Amsterdam: John Benjamins.

Nuyts, J. and Pederson, E. (1997) (eds.). *Language and Conceptualization*. Cambridge: Cambridge University Press.

O

O'Malley, J. M. and Chamot, A. U. (1990). *Learning Strategies in Second Language Acquisition*. Cambridge: Cambridge University Press.

Obler, L. K. (1980). Right Hemisphere Participation in Second Language Acquisition. In: K. Diller (ed.), *Individual Differences and Universals in Language Learning Aptitude*, 87-98. Rowley, Mass.: Newbury House.

Obler, L. K. (1983). Knowledge in Neuroscience: The Case of Bilingualism. *Language Learning* 33: 159-191.

Obler, L. K. (1988). Neuroscience and Parameter-Setting. In: S. Flynn and W. O'Neil (eds.), *Linguistics in Second Language Acquisition*, 117-126. Dordrecht: Kluwer.

Obler, L. K. and Gjerlow, K. (1999). *Language and the Brain*. Cambridge: Cambridge University Press.

Odlin, T. (1989). *Language Transfer*. Cambridge: Cambridge University Press.

Ogden, C. K. and Richards, I. A. (1923). *The Meaning of Meaning*. London: Routledge and Kegan Paul.

Ojemann, G. A. (1977). Subcortical Mechanism. In: H. A. Whitaker (ed.), *Studies in Neurolinguistics*, 106-134. New York: Academic.

Oller, J. W. (1993). *Methods that Work: Ideas for Literacy and Language Teachers*. Boston: Heinle and Heinle.

Omaggio, A. (1978). *Games and Simulations in the Foreign Language Classroom*. Washington, D. C.: Center for Applied Linguistics.

Omaggio, A. (1982). Using Games and Interactional Activities for the Development of Functional Proficiency in a Second Language. *Canadian Modern Language Review* 38: 515-546.

Omaggio, A. (1986). *Teaching Language in Context*. Boston: Heinle and Heinle.

Ombredane, A., Alajouanine, T., and Durand, M. (1939). *Le syndrome de désintégration phonétique dans l'aphasie*. Paris: Masson.

Opie, I. and Opie, P. (1959). *The Lore and Language of Schoolchildren*. Frogmore: Paladin.

Ornstein, R. E. (1997). *The Right Mind: Making Sense of the Hemispheres*. New York: Harcourt Brace.

Ortony, A. (1979) (ed.). *Metaphor and Thought*. Cambridge: Cambridge University Press.

Osgood, C. E. and Sebeok, T. A. (1954) (eds.). *Psycholinguistics: A Survey of Theory and Research Problems*. Baltimore: Waverley Press.

Osgood, C. E. and Suci, G. E. (1953). Factor Analysis of Meaning. *Journal of Experimental Psychology* 49: 325-328.

Ostrosky-Solis, F. (1984). Right-Hemisphere Function and Language Development: A Neuropsychological and Psycholinguistic Research Review. In: A. Ardila and F. Ostrosky-Solis (eds.), *The Right Hemisphere: Neurology and Neuropsychology*, 145-169. New York: Gordon and Breach.

Ostrove, J. M., Simpson, T., and Gardner, H. (1990). Beyond Scripts: A Note on the Capacity of Right-Hemisphere-Damaged Patients to Process Social and Emotional Content. *Brain and Cognition* 12: 144-154.

P

Paivio, A. (1979). Psychological Processes in the Comprehension of Metaphor. In: A. Ortony (ed.), *Metaphor and Thought*, 150-171. Cambridge: Cambridge University Press.

Pallotta, L. I. (1993). The "Bimodal" Aspect of Proficiency-Oriented Instruction. *Foreign Language Annals* 26: 429-434.

Palmer, A. and Rodgers, T. S. (1983). Games in Language Teaching. *Language Teaching* 16: 2-21.

Palmer, H. (1917). *The Scientific Teaching and Study of Languages*. Yonkers-on-Hudson: World Book.

Palmer, H. (1921). *The Oral Method of Teaching Languages*. Cambridge: Heffer.

Palmer, H. (1922). *The Principles of Language-Study*. Oxford: Oxford University Press.

Palmer, H. and Palmer, D. (1925). *English through Actions*. London: Longman.

Panther, K-U and Radden, G. (1999) (eds.). *Metonymy in Language and Thought*. Amsterdam: John Benjamins.

Paradis, M. (1987). *The Assessment of Bilingual Aphasia*. Hillsdale, N. J.: Lawrence Erlbaum.

Paradis, M., Hagiwara, H., and Hildbrandt, N. (1985). *Neurolinguistic Aspects of the Japanese Writing System*. New York: Academic.

Patterson, C. H. (1973). *Humanistic Education*. New Jersey: Prentice-Hall.

Peal, E. and Lambert, W. E. (1962). The Relation of Bilingualism to Intelligence. *Psychological Monographs* 76, Entire Issue.

Peirce, C. S. (1931-1958). *Collected Papers*. Cambridge: Harvard University Press.

Penfield, W. and Rasmussen, R. (1950). *The Cerebral Cortex of Man*. New York: Macmillan.

Penfield, W. and Roberts, H. (1959). *Speech and Brain Mechanisms*. Princeton: Princeton University Press.

Perecman, E. (1989). Language Processing in the Bilingual: Evidence from Language Mixing. In: K. Hiltenstam and L. K. Obler (eds.), *Bilingualism across the Lifespan*, 227-244. Cambridge: Cambridge University Press.

Piaget, J. (1923). *Le langage et la pensée chez l'enfant*. Neuchâtel: Delachaux et Niestlé.

Piaget, J. (1936). *L'intelligence avant le langage*. Paris: Flammarion.

Piaget, J. (1945). *La formation du symbole chez l'enfant*. Neuchâtel: Delachaux et Niestlé.

Piaget, J. (1955). *The Language and Thought of the Child*. Cleveland: Meredian.

Piaget, J. (1969). *The Child's Conception of the World*. Totowa: Littlefield, Adams and Company.

Pinker, S. (1990). Language Acquisition. In: D. N. Osherson and H. Lasnik (eds.), *Language: An Invitation to Cognitive Science*, 191-241. Cambridge: MIT Press.

Pinker, S. (1994). *The Language Instinct: How the Mind Creates Language*. New Tork: Morrow.

Piper, D. (1985). Contrastive Rhetoric and Reading in Second Language: Theoretical Perspectives on Classroom Practice. *Canadian Modern Language Review* 42: 34-43.

Polk, M. and Kertesz, A. (1993). Music and Language in Degenerative Disease of the Brain. *Brain and Cognition* 22: 98-117.

Pollio, H. and Burns, B. (1977). The Anomaly of Anomaly. *Journal of Psycholinguistic Research* 6: 247-260.

Pollio, H. and Smith, M. (1979). Sense and Nonsense in Thinking about Anomaly and Metaphor. *Bulletin of the Psychonomic Society* 13: 323-326.

Pollio, H., Barlow, J., Fine, H., and Pollio, M. (1977). T*he Poetics of Growth: Figurative Language in Psychology, Psychotherapy, and Education*. Hillsdale, N. J.: Lawrence Erlbaum Associates.

Pollio, H., Barrow, J., Fine, H., and Pollio, M. (1977). *Psychology and the Poetics of Growth: Figurative Language in Psychology, Psychotherapy, and Education*. Hillsdale, NJ: Lawrence Erlbaum Associates.

Porcelli, G. (1994). *Principi di glottodidattica*. Brescia: Editrice La Scuola.

Porter, R. P. (1990). *Forked Tongue: The Politics of Bilingual Education*. New York: Basic Books.

Potter, J. (1996). *Representing Reality: Discourse, Rhetoric, and Social Construction*. Thousand Oaks, Ca.: Sage Publications.

Poyatos, F. (1989). Nonverbal Communication in Foreign-language Teaching and Learning: A Theoretical and Methodological Approach. In: A. Helbo (ed.), *Evaluation and Language Teaching*, 45-59. Frankfurt: Peter Lang.

Propp, V. J. (1928). *Morphology of the Folktale*. Austin: University of Texas Press.

Pulvermueller, F. and Schumann, J. H. (1994). Neurological Mechanisms of Language Acquisition. *Language Learning* 44: 681-734.

R

Raffler-Engel, W. von (1980). Kinesics and Paralinguistics: A Neglected Factor in Second-Language Research and Teaching. *Canadian Modern Language Review* 36: 1980: 225-237.

Raina, M. K. (1984). *Education of the Left and the Right: Implications of Hemispheric Specialization*. New Delhi: Allied Publishers.

Ramírez, A. (1995). *Creating Context for Second Language Acquisition: Theory and Methods*. New York: Longman.

Rapcsak, S. Z., Beeson, P. M., and Rubens, A. B. (1991). Writing with the Right Hemisphere. *Brain and Language* 41: 510-530.

Rayman, J. and Zaidel, E. (1991). Rhyming and the Right Hemisphere. *Brain and Language* 40: 89-103.

Rector, M. and Trinta, A. R. (1985). *Comunicação não verbal: A gestualidade Brazileira*. Petropolis: Editor Vozes.

Ressler, L. E. (1991). Improving Elderly Recall with Bimodal Presentation: A Natural Experiment of Discharge Planning. *The Gerontologist* 31: 364-370.

Reynolds, A. G. (1992) (ed.). *Bilingualism, Multiculturalism, and Second Language Learning*. Hillsdale, N. J.: Lawrence Erlbaum Associates.

Richards, I. A. (1936). *The Philosophy of Rhetoric*. Oxford: Oxford University Press.

Richards, J. C. (1974) (ed.). *Error Analysis: Perspectives on Second Language Acquisition*. London: Longman.

Richards, J. C. (1975). Simplification: A Strategy in the Adult Acquisition of a Foreign Language. *Language Learning* 25: 115-126.

Richards, J. C. (1978) (ed.). *Second Language Acquisition*. Rowley, Mass.: Newbury House.

Richards, J. C. (1998). *Teaching in Action: Case Studies from Second Language Clasrooms*. Alexandria, Va.: Teachers of English to Speakers of Other Languages.

Richards, J. C. and Rodgers, T. S. (1986). *Approaches and Methods in Language Teaching: A Description and Analysis*. Cambridge: Cambridge University Press.

Richards, L. G. and Chiarello, C. (1989). Typicality Effects in Artificial Categories: Is There a Hemispheric Difference? *Brain and Language* 37: 90-106..

Richardson, I. M. (1989). Language and Humor. *British Journal of Language Teaching* 27: 142-147.

Richardson, J. T. E. (1991). Imagery and the Brain. In: C. Cornoldi and M. A. McDaniel (eds.), *Imagery and Cognition*, 1-31. New York: Springer.

Ridge, H. L. (1981). A Two-Way Street: Multiculturalism in Mathematics and Mathematics in Multiculturalism. In: K. A. McLeod (ed.), *Intercultural Education and Community Development*, 54-62. Toronto: University of Toronto Faculty of Education.

Ritchie, W. C. and Bhatia, T. (1996). Second Language Acquisition: Introduction, Foundations, and Overview. In: W. C. Ritchie and T. Bhatia (eds.), 1-46. *Handbook of Second Language Acquisition*. San Diego: Academic Press.

Ritchie, W. C. and Bhatia, T. K. (1996) (eds.). *Handbook of Second Language Acquisition*. San Diego: Academic Press.

Rivers, W. (1964). *The Psychologist and the Foreign Language Teacher*. Chicago: University of Chicago Press.

Rivers, W. (1983). *Communicating Naturally in a Second Language. Theory and Practice in Language Teaching*. Cambridge: Cambridge University Press.

Rixon, S. (1981). *How to Use Games in Language Teaching*. London: Macmillan.

Robinett, B. W. and Schachter, J. (1983) (eds.). *Second Language Learning: Contrastive Analysis, Error Analysis and Related Aspects*. Ann Arbor: University of Michigan Press.

Rodgers, T. S. (1981). A Framework for Making and Using Language Teaching Games. In: *Guidelines for Language Games*, 1-7. Singapore: RELC.

Rogers, C. (1951). *Client-Centered Therapy*. Boston: Houghton Mifflin.

Rogers, C. (1961). *On Becoming a Person: A Therapist's View of Psychotherapy*. Boston: Houghton Mifflin.

Rosch E. (1973a). On the Internal Structure of Perceptual and Semantic Categories. In: T. E. Moore (ed.), *Cognitive Development and Acquisition of Language*., 111-144. New York: Academic.

Rosch E. (1973b). Natural Categories. *Cognitive Psychology* 4: 328-350.

Rosch E. (1975a). Cognitive Reference Points. *Cognitive Psychology* 7: 532-547.

Rosch E. (1975b). Cognitive Representations of Semantic Categories. *Journal of Experimental Psychology* 104: 192-233.

Ross, E. D. and Mesulam, M. M. (1979). Dominant Language Functions of the Right Hemisphere: Prosody end Emotional Gesturing. *Archives of Neurology* 36: 144-148.

Rumelhart D. E. and McClelland, J. L. (1986) (eds.). *Parallel Distributed Processing*. Cambridge, Mass.: MIT Press.

Russo, G. A. (1997). *A Conceptual Fluency Framework for the Teaching of Italian as a Second Language*. Dissertation, University of Toronto.

S

Saer, D. J. (1923). The Effects of Bilingualism on Intelligence. *British Journal of Psychology* 14: 25-38.

Salvi, R. (1990). Strategie didattiche e applicazioni tecnologiche nell'insegnamento linguistico. *Scuola e Lingue Moderne* 28: 134-143.

Sapir, E. (1921). *Language*. New York: Harcourt, Brace, and World.

Satz, P., Strauss, E., and Whitaker, H. (1990). The Ontogeny of Hemispheric Specialization: Some Old Hypotheses Revisited. *Brain and Language* 38: 596-614.

Saussure, F. de (1916). *Cours de linguistique générale*. Paris: Payot.

Savignon, S. J. (1992). Problem Solving and the Negotiation of Meaning. In: C. Cicogna, M. Danesi, and A. Mollica (eds.), *Problem Solving in Second Language Teaching*, 11-25. Welland: Soleil.

Sawyers, J. K. and Rogers, C. S. (1994). *Helping Children Develop through Play*. Washington: National Association for the Education of Young Children.

Sayce, A. (1900). *Introduction to the Science of Language*. London: Kegan Paul, Trench, Trübner and Co.

Schacter, D. L. (1987). Implicit Memory: History and Current Status. *Journal of Experimental Psychology: Learning, Memory, and Cognition* 13: 501-508.

Schenone, P. (1994). Emisfero destro ed elaborazione linguistica, conferme e sollecitazioni per il modello didattico bimodale. *L'Analisi Linguistica e Letteraria* 2: 467-498.

Scherer, G. A. C. and Wertheimer, M. (1964). *A Psycholinguistic Experiment in Foreign-Language Teaching*. New York: McGraw-Hill.

Schiffler, L. (1992). *Suggestopedic Methods and Applications*. Philadelphia: Gordon and Breach Science Publishers.

Schloss, B. (1977). *Jeux linguistiques*. Toronto: OISE.

Schmidt, E. (1977). *Let's Play Games in German.* Skokie: National Textbook Co.

Schmitt, N. (2000). *Vocabulary in Language Teaching.* Cambridge: Cambridge University Press.

Schogt, H. (1988). *Linguistics, Literary Analysis, and Literary Translation.* Toronto: University of Toronto Press.

Schultz, M. and Fisher, A. (1988). *Games for All Reasons: Interacting in the Language Classroom.* Reading: Addison-Wesley.

Schulz, R. A. (1986). From Achievement to Proficiency through Classroom Instruction: Some Caveats. *Modern Language Journal* 70: 373-379

Schulz, R. A. (1991). Second Language Acquisition Theories and Teaching Practice: How Do They Fit? *Modern Language Journal* 75: 17-26.

Schumann, J. H. (1990). The Role of the Amygdala as a Mediator of Affect and Cognition in Second Language Acquisition. In: J. E. Alatis (ed.), *Proceedings of the Georgetown University Round Table on Language and Linguistics*, 169-176. Washington, D. C.: Georgetown University Press.

Schumann, J. H. and Jacobs, B. (1992). Language Acquisition and the Neurosciences: Towards a More Integrative Perspective. *Applied Linguistics* 13: 282-301.

Schwartz, G. E., Davidson, R. J., and Maer, F. (1975). Right Hemisphere Lateralization for Emotion in the Human Brain: Interactions with Cognition. *Science* 120: 286-288.

Scovel, T. (1982). Questions Concerning the Applicability of Neurolinguistic Research to Second Language Learning and Teaching. *TESOL Quarterly* 16: 323-332.

Scovel, T. (1988). *A Time to Speak: A Psycholinguistic Inquiry into the Critical Period for Human Speech.* Rowley, Mass.: Newbury House.

Scovel, T. (1998). *Psycholinguistics.* Oxford: Oxford University Press.

Searle, J. R. (1969). *Speech Acts: An Essay in the Philosophy of Language.* Cambridge: Cambridge University Press.

Searleman, A. A. (1977). Review of Right Hemisphere Linguistic Capabilities. *Psychological Bulletin* 84: 503-528.

Sebeok, T. A. (1976). *Contributions to the Doctrine of Signs.* Lanham: University Press of America.

Sebeok, T. A. (1979). *The Sign and Its Masters.* Austin: University of Texas Press.

Sebeok, T. A. (1981). *The Play of Musement.* Bloomington: Indiana University Press.

Sebeok, T. A. (1986). *I Think I Am a Verb: More Contributions to the Doctrine of Signs.* New York: Plenum.

Sebeok, T. A. (1991). *A Sign Is Just a Sign.* Bloomington: Indiana University Press.

Sebeok, T. A. (1994). *Signs: An Introduction to Semiotics.* Toronto: University of Toronto Press.

Sebeok, T. A. and Danesi, M. (2000). *The Forms of Meaning: Modeling Systems Theory and Semiotics.* Berlin: Mouton de Gruyter.

Seedhouse, P. (1994). Linking Pedagogical Purpose to Linguistic Patterns of Interaction: the Analysis of Communication in the Language Classroom. *International Review of Applied Linguistics* 32: 303-320.

Segalowitz, S. J. (1983). *Two Sides of the Brain: Brain Lateralization Explored.* Englewood Cliffs, N. J.: Prentice-Hall.

Segalowitz, S. S. and Cohen, H. (1989). Right Hemisphere Sensitivity to Speech. *Brain and Language* 37: 220-231.

Segalowitz. S. and Gruber, F. A. (1977). Some Issues and Methods in the Neuropsychology of Language. In: S. Segalowitz and F. A. Gruber (eds.), *Language Development and Neurological Theory*, 1-13. New York: Academic.

Seliger, H. (1978). Implications of a Multiple Critical Periods Hypothesis for Second Language Learning. In: W. Ritchie (ed.), *Second Language Acquisition Research*, 21-35. New York: Academic.

Seliger, H. (1980). On the Possible Role of the Right Hemisphere in Second Language Acquisition. *TESOL Quarterly* 16: 307-314.

Selinker, L. (1972). Interlanguage. *International Review of Applied Linguistics* 10: 209-231.

Shibles, W. (1989). How German Vocabulary Pictures Emotion. *British Journal of Language Teaching* 27: 141.

Shibles, W. (1989). How German Vocabulary Pictures Emotion. *British Journal of Language Teaching* 27: 141.

Shrum, J. L. and Glisan, E. W. (1994). *Contextualized Language Instruction.* Boston: Heinle and Heinle.

Singleton, D. (1989). *Language Acquisition: The Age Factor.* Clevedon: Multilingual Matters.

Singleton, D. (1999). *Exploring the Second Language Mental Lexicon.* Canbridge: Cambridge University Press.

Singleton, D. and Lengyel, Z. (1995) (eds.). *The Age Factor in Second Language Acquisition: A Critical Look at the Critical Period Hypothesis.* Clevedon: Multilingual Matters.

Skehan, P. (1998). *A Cognitive Approach to Language Learning.* Oxford: Oxford University Press.

Skinner, B. F. (1957). *Verbal Behavior.* New York: Appleton-Century-Crofts.

Skousen, R. (1989). *Analogical Modeling of Language.* Dordrecht: Kluwer.

Smith, F. (1923). Bilingualism and Mental Development. *British Journal of Psychology* 13: 271-282.

Smith, M. E. (1931). A Study of Five Bilingual Children from the Same Family. *Child Language* 2: 184-187.

Smith, M. E. (1939). Some Light on the Problem of Bilingualism as Found from a Study of the Progress in Mastery in English among Pre-School Children of Non-American Ancestry in Hawaii. *Genetic Psychology Monographs* 21: 119-284.

Smith, P. D. (1970). *A Comparison of the Cognitive and Audio-Lingual Approaches to Foreign Language Instruction.* Philadelphia: Center for Curriculum Development.

Smor Foster, E. (1995). *The Role of Cognitive Lateral Eye Movement as an Indicator of Cognitive Activity during Mental Processing in a Structured L1 and L2 Learning Environment.* Dissertation, Ontario Institute for Studies in Education.

Snow, M. A. and Brinton, D. (1997) (eds.), *The Content-Based Classroom: Perspectives on Integrating Language and Content.* New York: Longman.

Solso, R. L. (1997) (ed.). *Mind and Brain Sciences in the 21st Century.* Cambridge, Mass.: MIT Press.

Sontag, S. (1978). *Illness as Metaphor.* New York: Farrar, Straus and Giroux.

Sontag, S. (1989). *AIDS and Its Metaphors.* New York: Farrar, Straus and Giroux.

Sousa, D. A. (1998). *Learning Manual for How the Brain Learns.* Thousand Oaks, Ca.: Corwin Press.

Sperry, R. W. (1968). Hemisphere Disconnection and Unity in Conscious Awareness. *American Psychologist* 23: 723-733.

Sperry, R. W. (1968). Hemisphere Disconnection and Unity in Conscious Awareness. *American Psychologist* 23: 723-733.

Sperry, R. W. (1973). Lateral Specialization of Cerebral Function in the Surgically Separated Hemisphere. In: P. J. Vinken and G. W. Bruyn (eds.), *The Psychophysiology of Thinking,* 273-289. Amsterdam: North Holland.

Spolsky, B. (1985). Formulating a Theory of Second Language Learning. *Studies in Second Language Acquisition* 7: 269-288.

Spolsky, B. (1989). *Conditions for Second Language Learning.* Oxford: Oxford University Press.

Spolsky, B. (1998). *Sociolinguistics.* Oxford: Oxford University Press.

Springer, S. P. and Deutsch, G. (1993). *Left Brain, Right Brain.* New York: W. H. Freeman.

Sridhar, S. N. (1981). Contrastive Analysis, Error Analysis and Interlanguage: Three Phases of One Goal. In: J. Fisiak (ed.), *Contrastive Linguistics and the Language Teacher,* 207-241. Oxford: Pergamon.

Stachowiak, F., Huber, W., Poeck, K., and Kerschensteiner, M. (1977). Text Comprehension in Aphasia. *Brain and Language* 4: 177-195.

Staehlin, W. (1914). Zür Psychologie und Statistike der Metapherm. *Archiv für Gesamte Psychologie* 31, 299-425.

Steinberg, J. (1991). *Games Language People Play.* Markham: Dominie Press.

Stern, H. H. (1983) *Fundamental Concepts of Language Teaching*. Oxford: Oxford University Press.

Stevick, E. W. (1976). *Memory, Meaning and Method. Some Psychological Perspectives on Language Learning*. Rowley Mass.: Newbury House Publishers.

Stevick, E. W. (1980). *Teaching Language. A Way and Ways*. Rowley Mass.: Newbury House Publishers.

Stevick, E. W. (1990). *Humanism in Language Teaching*. Oxford: Oxford University Press.

Stieblich, C. (1983). *Language Learning: A Study on Cognitive Style, Lateral Eye-Movement and Deductive vs. Inductive Learning of Foreign Language Structures*. Dissertation, McGill University, Montreal.

Stockwell, R. P., Bowen, D. J., and Martin, J. W. (1965a). *The Sounds of English and Spanish*. Chicago: University of Chicago Press.

Stockwell, R. P., Bowen, D. J., and Martin, J. W. (1965b). *The Grammatical Structures of English and Spanish*. Chicago: University of Chicago Press.

Sweet, H. (1899). *The Practical Study of Languages: A Guide for Teachers and Learners*. London: J. M. Dent & Sons.

Sweetser, E. (1990). *From Etymology to Pragmatics: The Mind-as-Body Metaphor in Semantic Structure and Semantic Change*. Cambridge: Cambridge University Press.

T

Taggart, W. and Torrance, E. P. (1984). *Human Information Processing Survey*. Bensenville, Ill.: Scholastic Testing Service.

Tannen, D. (1989). *Talking Voices*. Cambridge: Cambridge University Press.

Taylor, J. R. (1995). *Linguistic Categorization: Prototypes in Linguistic Theory*. Oxford: Oxford University Press.

Temple, C. (1993). *The Brain: An Introduction to the Psychology of the Human Brain and Behaviour*. Harmondsworth: Penguin.

Terrell, T. D. (1991). The Role of Grammar Instruction in a Communicative Approach. *Modern Language Journal* 75: 52-63.

Thomas, M. (1995). Medieval and Modern Views of Universal Grammar and the Nature of Second Language Learning. *Modern Language Journal* 79: 345-355.

Titone, R. (1968). *Teaching Foreign Languages: An Historical Sketch*. Washington, D. C.: Georgetown University Press.

Titone, R. and Danesi, M. (1985). *Applied Psycholinguistics: An Introduction to the Psychology of Second Language Learning and Teaching*. Toronto: University of Toronto Press.

Tollefson, J. W., Jacobs, B., and Selipsky, E. (1977). The Monitor Model and Neurofunctional Theory: An Integrated View. *Studies in Second Language Acquisition* 6: 1-16.

Tosi, A. (1984). *Immigration and Bilingual Education*. Oxford: Pergamon.

Travis, L. (1988). Linguistic Theory: Neuroscience and Second Language Acquisition. In: S. Flynn and W. O'Neil (eds.), *Linguistics in Second Language Acquisition*, 90-108. Dordrecht: Kluwer.

Trevarthen, C. (1990) (ed.). *Brain Circuits and Functions of the Mind: Essays in Honor of Roger W. Sperry*. Cambridge: Cambridge University Press.

Turner, M. (1996). *The Literary Mind: The Origins of Thought and Language*. Oxford: Oxford University Press.

U

Unterbeck, B., Rissanen, M., Nevelainen, T., and Saari, M. (1999). *Gender in Grammar and Cognition*. Berlin: Mouton de Gruyter.

V

Vaid, J. (1983). Bilingualism and Brain Lateralization. In: S. J. Segalowitz (ed.), *Language Functions and Brain Lateralization*, 315-340. New York: Academic Press.

Vaid, J. and Genesee, F. (1980). Neuropsychological Approaches to Bilingualism: A Critical Review. *Canadian Journal of Psychology* 34: 419-447.

Vaid, J. and Hall, J. D. (1991). Neuropsychological Perspectives on Bilingualism: Right, Left, and Center. In: A. G. Reynolds (eds.), *Bilingualism, Multiculturalism, and Second Language Learning*, 81-112. Hillsdale, N. J.: Lawrence Erlbaum Associates.

Valdman, A. (1961). *Applied Linguistics: French*. Boston: D. C. Heath.

Valdman, A. (1966) (ed.). *Trends in Language Teaching*. New York: McGraw-Hill.

Valdman, A. (1975). Error Analysis and Grading in the Preparation of Teaching Material. *Modern Language Journal* 59: 422-426.

Valdman, A. (1995). Classroom Language Learning Research: Reliability and Applicability. *Il Forneri* 9: 42-58.

Valdman, A. (2001). *Essays in Applied Linguistics*. Ottawa: Legas.

Valdman, A. and Pons, C. (1997). *Chez nous: Branché sur le monde francophone*. Upper Sadle River: Prentice Hall.

Van de Craen, P. (1990). Allochthonous Minorities and Contact Linguistics: Towards a Language Learning Paradigm Based on Social Linguistic Principles. *Sociolinguistica* 4: 98-112.

Van Dijk, T. (1997) (ed.). *Discourse as Social Interaction*. London: Sage.

Van Ek, J. A. (1975). *The Threshold Level in a European Unit/Credit System for Modern Language Teaching by Adults*. Strasbourg: Council of Europe.

Vargha-Khadem, F. et al. (1997). Onset of Speech After Left Hemisperectomy in a Nine-Year-Old Boy. *Brain* 120: 159-182.

Verhoeven, L. T. (1994). Transfer in Bilingual Development: The Linguistic Intedependence Hypothesis Revisited», *Language Learning* 44: 381-415.

Viëtor, W. (1882). *Der Sprachunterricht muss umkerhren! Ein Beitrag zur Uberündungsfrages*. Heilbronn.

Vining, E. P. G. et al. (1997). Why Would You Remove Half a Brain? The Outcome of 58 Children After Hemisperectomy—The Johns Hopkins Experience: 1968 to 1996. *Pediatrics* 100: 163-171.

Vygotsky, L. S. (1962). *Thought and Language*. Cambridge, Mass.: MIT Press.

Vygotsky, L. S. (1978). *Mind in Society*. Cambridge, Mass.: Cambridge University Press.

W

Walker, J. (1990). Of Brains and Rhetorics. *College English* 52: 301-322.

Walsh, T. and Diller, K. (1978). Neurolinguistic Foundation to Methods of Teaching a Second Language. *International Review of Applied Linguistics* 16: 1-14.

Walsh, T. and Diller, K. (1981). Neurolinguistic Considerations on the Optimum Age for Second Language Learning. In: K. Diller (ed.), *Universals in Language Learning Aptitude*, 34-45. Rowley, Mass.: Newbury House.

Wapner, W., Hamby, S., and Gardner, H. (1981). The Role of the Right Hemisphere in the Apprehension of Complex Linguistic Materials. *Brain and Language* 14: 15-33.

Wardhaugh, R. (1970). The Contrastive Analysis Hypothesis. *TESOL Quarterly* 4: 123-130.

Way, E. C. (1991). *Knowledge Representation and Metaphor*. Dordrecht: Kluwer.

Weber-Fox, C. M. and Neville, H. J. (1996). Maturational Constraints on Functional Specializations for Language Processing: ERP and Behavioral Evidence in Bilingual Speakers. *Journal of Cognitive Neuroscience* 8: 231-256.

Webster, M. and Castonon, E. (1980). *Crosstalk: Communication Tasks and Games at the Elementary, Preintermediate and Intermediate Levels*. Oxford: Oxford University Press.

Weinstein, E. A. (1964). Affections of Speech with Lesions of the Non-Dominant Hemisphere. *Research Publications of the Association for Research on Nervous and Mental Disorders* 42: 220-225.

Weisler, S. E. and Milekic, S. (2000). *Theory of Language*. Cambridge, Mass." MIT Press.

Wells, G. (1986). *The Meaning Makers: Children Learning Language and Using Language to Learn.* Portsmouth: Heinemann.

Wernicke, C. (1874). *Der aphasische Symptomenkomplex*. Breslau: Cohn and Weigart.

Whitaker, H. A. (1992). Lateralization of Language. In: W. Bright (ed.), *International Encyclopedia of Linguistics*, vol. 2, 310-313. Oxford: Oxford University Press.

White, L. (1989). *Universal Grammar and Second Language Acquisition.* Amsterdam: John Benjamins.

White, L. (1990) Second Language Acquisition and Universal Grammar. *Studies in Second Language Acquisition* 12: 121-133.

White. L. (1989). *Universal Grammar and Second Language Acquisition.* Amsterdam: John Benjamins.

Whorf, B. L. (1956). *Language, Thought and Reality.* Cambridge, Mass.: MIT Press.

Widdowson, H. G (1972). *Teaching Language as Communication.* Oxford: Oxford University Press.

Wierzbicka, A. (1996). *Semantics: Primes and Universals*. Oxford: Oxford University Press.

Wilkins, D. A. (1976). *Notional Syllabuses.* Oxford: Oxford University Press.

Wilkinson, J. A. (1993). Drama, Brain and Meaning. In: J. A. Wilkinson (ed.), *The Symbolic Dramatic Play-Literacy Connection: Whole Brain, Whole Body, Holistic Learning*, 59-68. Needham Heights, Mass.: Ginn.

Willis, J. (1996). *A Framework for Task-Based Learning*. London: Longman.

Winner, E. (1979). New Names for Old Things: The Emergence of Metaphoric Language. *Journal of Child Language* 6: 469-492.

Winner, E. (1982). Invented Worlds: The Psychology of the Arts. Cambridge: Harvard University Press.

Winner, E. (1988). *The Point of Words: Children's Understanding of Metaphor and Irony*. Cambridge, Mass.: Harvard University Press.

Winner, E. and Gardner, H. (1977). The Comprehension of Metaphor in Brain-Damaged Patients. *Brain* 100: 717-729.

Witelson, S. F. (1977). Early Hemisphere Specialization and Interhemisphere Plasticity: An Empirical and Theoretical Review. In: S. J. Segalowitz and F. A. Gruber (eds.), *Language Development and Neurological Theory*, 214-257. New York: Academic.

Wode, H. (1976). Developmental Sequences in Naturalistic L2 Acquisition. *Working Papers in Bilingualism* 11: 1-13.

Wolfe, D. E. (1972). Teacher-Made Crossword Puzzles. *Audio-Visual Language Journal* 10: 177-181.

Wolff, D. (1987). Some Assumptions about Second Language Text Comprehension. *Studies in Second Language Acquisition* 9: 307-326.

Wright, A., Betteridge, D. and Buckby, M. (1979). *Games for Language Learning*. Cambridge: Cambridge University Press.

Wuillemin, D., Richardson, B., and Lynch, J. (1994). Right Hemisphere Involvement in Processing Later-Learned Languages in Multilinguals. *Brain and Language* 46: 620-636.

Y

Yoshioka, J. G. (1929). A Study of Bilingualism *Journal of Genetic Psychology* 36: 473-479.

Yu, N. (1998). *The Contemporary Theory of Metaphor: A Perspective from Chinese*. Amsterdam: John Benjamins.

Yule, G. (1996). *Pragmatics*. Cambridge: Cambridge University Press.

Z

Zaidel, E. (1983). On Multiple Representations of the Lexicon in the Brain: The Case of Two Hemispheres. In: M. Studdert-Kennedy (ed.), *Psychobiology of Language,* 105-125. Cambridge, Mass.: MIT Press.

Zaidel, E., White, H., Sakurai, E., and Banks, W. (1988). Hemispheric Locus of Lexical Congruity Effects: Neuropsychological Reinterpretation of Psycholinguistic Results. In: C. Chiarello (ed.), *Right Hemisphere Contributions to Lexical Semantics,* 71-87. New York: Springer.

Zatorre, R. J. (1989). On the Representation of Multiple Languages in the Brain: Old Problems and New Directions. *Brain and Language* 36: 127-147

Zobl, H. (1995). Converging Evidence for the "Acquisition-Learning" Distinction. *Applied Linguistics* 16: 35-55.

INDEX